HEART
TO
HEART

v

*A Cleveland Clinic Guide
to Understanding Heart Disease
and Open Heart Surgery*

HEART
TO
HEART

by **NORMAN V. RICHARDS**
*With Assistance by Staff Members
of The Cleveland Clinic Foundation*

Introduction by Floyd D. Loop, M.D.
Chairman, Department of Thoracic
and Cardiovascular Surgery
The Cleveland Clinic Foundation

ATHENEUM
1987
NEW YORK

Library of Congress Cataloging-in-Publication Data
Richards, Norman.
  Heart to heart.
    1. Aortocoronary bypass. 2. Heart—Diseases—Popular
works. 3. Cleveland Clinic Foundation. I. Cleveland
Clinic Foundation. II. Title.
RD598.R49 1987   617'.412   86-47694
ISBN 0-689-11854-6

Copyright © 1987 by Norman V. Richards
All rights reserved
Published simultaneously in Canada by Collier Macmillan Canada, Inc.
Composition by Maryland Linotype Composition Company,
  Baltimore, Maryland
Manufactured by Fairfield Graphics, Fairfield, Pennsylvania
Designed by Laura Rohrer
First Edition

TO ROBIN,
WITH MY LOVE
AND ADMIRATION

Acknowledgments

I am deeply grateful for the cooperation given to me by the people of the Cleveland Clinic Foundation, one of the world's leading medical institutions.

First, to William S. Kiser, M.D., Chairman of the Board of Governors, who agreed with my idea that a book written by a former Cleveland Clinic heart surgery patient could help other patients and their families understand heart disease and open heart surgery better.

Thanks are also due the renowned surgeon Floyd D. Loop, M.D., and the superb staff he heads as Chairman of the Department of Thoracic and Cardiovascular Surgery, including Delos Cosgrove, M.D., who performed my own coronary bypass surgery, and Paul Taylor, M.D., who allowed me to observe two entire open heart operations as he described the procedures to me.

I am also grateful to Earl K. Shirey, M.D., the highly respected cardiologist who has been my doctor at the Cleveland Clinic since my surgery. Dr. Shirey kindly consented to answer my many questions at interviews and to review the manuscript of this book.

My thanks, too, to the skilled, dedicated professionals of the operating room staff, the nursing staff, the technicians, and others who took time to explain their jobs to me, as well as the public affairs professionals who helped to arrange my interviews and provided photography and art for this book. If this book proves to be helpful to heart patients, all these people deserve the credit.

NORMAN V. RICHARDS

Introduction

In medicine's long march of progress in treating heart disease, few developments have had such an impact as open heart surgery. It has been less than two decades since coronary artery bypass surgery was developed by Rene G. Favaloro, M.D., at the Cleveland Clinic Foundation. In that short time span, it has become the most frequent cardiac operation worldwide. Approximately 200,000 coronary bypass operations are performed in the United States annually.

There are four treatment modalities directed at coronary atherosclerosis: beta-blocking drugs, calcium antagonists, balloon angioplasty, and coronary bypass surgery. Coronary artery bypass surgery has been scrutinized more than any other treatment. Numerous retrospective and prospective studies have shown conclusively that surgery relieves angina more dramatically and more consistently than medical treatment. Extensive experience with this procedure has demonstrated that improving blood supply to the heart muscle reduces symptoms and restores more normal exercise tolerance. Now there is evidence that the operation improves longevity in patients with high-risk coronary artery disease and reduces the frequency of later cardiac hospitalizations, subsequent heart attacks, and sudden death. To many patients, this surgery represents a second chance for an active, pain-free life.

Coronary artery bypass surgery is not curative and does not arrest or even retard the ongoing process of atherosclerosis. Furthermore, surgery cannot reverse the permanent effect that a heart attack has had on the heart muscle. Each patient's case should be evaluated individually; surgery is not an automatic choice of treatment in all cases of coronary atherosclerosis. Many diagnostic technologies are now available to determine the best treatment during the course of the disease.

One of the more hopeful developments in combating coronary artery disease in recent years has been a growing public awareness of the risk factors associated with the disease. A considerable body of evidence has been compiled showing that such factors as cigarette smoking, diets rich in cholesterol and saturated fats, obesity, hypertension, and lack of exercise are associated with increased risk of coronary artery disease. We have seen a significant decline in mortality from heart disease over the past two decades in this country, and while we lack conclusive proof for the reasons, the decline coincides with a greater public inclination to refrain from smoking, eating high-fat foods, and following sedentary lifestyles. Prevention is likely to play a large role in further declines of heart disease mortality.

Heart patients, including those who have had open heart surgery, can be helpful to other patients by aiding them in understanding heart disease. Norman Richards had that goal in mind when he wrote this book with

Introduction

the aid of staff physicians at the Cleveland Clinic Foundation.

Shortly after he learned that he had coronary artery disease, Mr. Richards underwent coronary artery bypass surgery at the Cleveland Clinic in 1982. His lack of knowledge about atherosclerosis convinced him that he should learn as much as possible about the disease and adopt lifestyle changes to reduce his risk factors. In this book, he discusses heart disease in plain English, and describes the risk factors associated with it, diagnostic procedures and treatment, and the details of coronary artery bypass surgery.

FLOYD D. LOOP, M.D.
Chairman, Department of Thoracic
and Cardiovascular Surgery
The Cleveland Clinic Foundation

Contents

ONE	*A Case of Heart Disease*	3
TWO	*Nature's Marvelous Pump*	32
THREE	*Heart Disease: What Goes Wrong with the Pump*	39
FOUR	*Look at Your Risk Factors*	52
FIVE	*Diagnosing Heart Problems*	91
SIX	*Should You Have Surgery?*	106
SEVEN	*Preparing for Surgery*	118
EIGHT	*Open Heart Surgery*	127
NINE	*The Intensive Care Unit*	155
TEN	*Striving for Full Recovery*	167
ELEVEN	*Adopting a New, Healthier Life-Style*	183
TWELVE	*What's Ahead in Treating Heart Disease*	200
GLOSSARY		215

HEART
TO
HEART

1.
A Case of Heart Disease

UNSEEN, unfelt, coronary heart disease occurs insidiously in the otherwise healthy bodies of unsuspecting people. A typical victim, like the author of this book, is profoundly shocked to learn that he or she has anything as serious as heart disease.

My discovery came in December of 1981, when I was 49 years old. Two years earlier, I had accepted a very good offer to become manager of Marathon Oil Company's publications department in the pleasant, small city of Findlay, Ohio. Part of the job's appeal was a less stressful, less tiring life than the big-city commuter's existence I had led for years while working in New York City and living in Connecticut. Indeed Findlay does offer a more relaxed life-style than big cities, but it does not guarantee a stress-free life to any individual. In fact, I experienced a good deal of stress during my first two years in Findlay. In addition to my adjustments to a new job and a new community, I faced the end of a marriage that could not survive these adjustments. Then in the fall of 1981 came a threat to the existence of Marathon Oil and the economic well-being of Findlay. Mobil Corporation mounted an aggressive campaign to buy up Marathon's stock and merge the company into its own larger organization. Thousands of Marathon employees would lose their jobs and the city of Findlay, in losing its largest employer, would be economically devastated. As Marathon's management fought the Mobil takeover in the courts, in the news media, and in the financial arena, we in the company's press and publications organization were working nights, and weekends, and sometimes twenty-four hours straight, to put out special publications and other messages to employees and to the public. The stress and worry reached very high levels during this time—not only for us, but for all the company's employees and their families, as well as other townspeople.

Despite the stress in my life, I didn't give a thought to my health at that time. I had always been an exceptionally healthy person; I was one of those people who never got sick, or even caught colds. I have a strong, muscular body (which too easily gains weight when I don't watch my calories) and I've always felt vigorous and energetic.

As a professional writer and editor, and as an avid reader, I should have been much more aware of the risk factors in heart disease than I was in 1981. But like most ostensibly healthy people, I thought heart disease was something that happened to others. Sure, I was aware of a history of heart disease in my family. My father had

1. A Case of Heart Disease

angina pains for more than three decades before he died of a heart attack at the age of seventy-three. His brothers and sisters died of the same disease. But I didn't know then how important a family history of heart disease is as a risk factor.

I was aware of other risk factors: smoking, lack of exercise, improper diet. But I didn't give them much thought. I had never smoked cigarettes, although I had been an all-day-long pipe smoker for twenty-five years. I had always been fairly active, walking a mile or two every day in New York like many commuters, playing a little tennis, hiking on country roads, and cross-country skiing in my spare time. But I didn't know anything about the requirements of aerobic exercise and cardiovascular conditioning; my recreational exercise was done sporadically as fun with my wife and children, and I had no regular schedule for it. In the matter of diet, I had always indulged in my favorite foods: bacon and egg breakfasts; ice cream, cake, and pie; steak and french fries. I knew these were high in cholesterol and saturated fats, but I told myself that I consumed them in moderation. In fact, my serum cholesterol levels were reported on the high side of normal in my annual physical examinations, but they weren't quite high enough to elicit warnings from the examining physicians.

In November 1981, a few days after Mobil launched its threat to my job security, I passed my annual physical examination with flying colors, as I always did. My primary physician in Findlay, Dr. Gary Hirschfeld, conducted the examination and reported that, in general, I appeared to be quite healthy. He summarized, "This is a pleasant, mildly overweight white male in no acute distress." He did note that my biochemical profile showed a mild elevation of triglycerides (blood fats) at 226; high normal is 175. My cholesterol was in the normal range, although the high density lipoprotein (HDL) fraction of my total cholesterol was a little lower than optimum at 38. There was nothing on the electrocardiogram to cause alarm. Dr. Hirschfeld summarized his recommendations: "This patient is in overall excellent health. I advised him that he may benefit by some weight reduction. I would expect his triglycerides would decline also. His coronary risk factors are really quite low. He will consider returning to a regular exercise program in hopes of improving the HDL fraction somewhat."

Having my belief in my vigorous health confirmed once again, I plunged into the hectic situation at work as my company pursued its ferocious struggle to ward off Mobil's threat to its existence. Four weeks after my physical, in early December, I began to experience dull pains in my chest during my two-mile walks after dinner. I noticed that the pain radiated to both my upper arms as I walked. I remembered that my father had described his angina pains as "feeling like a toothache in the arms," and I noticed that the pain didn't last more than four or five minutes. As I continued walking, it would go away. But it returned nearly every time I walked. Finally I noticed that it occurred even in the mornings as I walked to my office from the parking lot.

1. A Case of Heart Disease

My ex-wife and grown children came to Ohio to celebrate a family Christmas at my house that year. Preparing for their arrival, I chopped a good-sized load of wood for the fireplace and carried many armloads of it into the house. The pain in my chest and arms was more severe than usual as I worked. By now, three weeks after I had noticed the pain, I was getting worried that it might be angina.

I didn't mention the pain to my family because I didn't want to worry them and diminish the happy feelings we all had at Christmas. But as soon as their holiday visit was over, I called Dr. Hirschfeld's office for an appointment. It was December 31, New Year's Eve, and I planned to go to dinner and to a party with some friends. Dr. Hirschfeld saw me that day and arranged a treadmill stress test in the offices of his group practice.

I was feeling fine as I prepared to step onto the motorized treadmill. I had worried over the possibility of having angina confirmed, but part of me believed this test would show that I had no cause for concern after all. Dr. Hirschfeld administered the test himself, assisted by a nurse who attached a number of electrodes to my chest. He explained the test procedures, pointing out that most people are able to walk for nine or ten minutes on the machine, at gradually increasing speeds and uphill grades, when there are no positive findings. The objective is to observe the heart's function on an electrocardiogram as the heart rate increases to a predetermined maximum.

The treadmill started moving, and I began walking confidently. I was told to let the doctor and nurse know if I felt any pain, but I felt so vigorous that I doubted I would have any. In stage one of the test, at the slowest speed and least incline, I felt fine. This stage lasts three minutes. After I assured him that I felt no pain, Dr. Hirschfeld began stage two, at a slightly increased speed and incline. Immediately, I began to feel a very slight, dull ache in my chest, which quickly progressed to a definite, more pronounced ache. At the same time, the electrocardiogram was recording changes in the way my heart was functioning, in the form of ST segment depressions. After only one and one-half minutes of stage two, the doctor halted the test and told me to sit down. As he observed the electrocardiogram, my ST segment changes moved toward normal very quickly. However, a few minutes after the exercise was halted, my heart rate began fluctuating between fifty and ninety-four beats a minute, in what is called arrhythmia. I was given a nitroglycerin tablet to dissolve under my tongue, and the arrhythmia subsided within two minutes.

What did the test result mean? Dr. Hirschfeld stated in his report for my medical record: "Abnormal stress test. This patient exercised for a total of 4.5 minutes, achieving a maximum heart rate of 140, which is just 75 percent of his predicted maximum. The test was terminated because of development of dull anterior chest pain and ischemic ST segment changes.... In summary, then, this stress test demonstrated very definite ischemic ST segment changes in both V5 and AVF leads at a very low

1. A Case of Heart Disease

work load, indicative of ischemic heart disease." (*Ischemia* is defined as a lack of oxygen in an organ or a tissue.)

"This test gives a strong indication that there is some obstruction of the blood flow to some part of your heart," Dr. Hirschfeld told me. "It looks as though you have some coronary artery blockage, and it could be severe. The most accurate method of determining which arteries are obstructed and to what extent is coronary angiography."

I had heard of this remarkable diagnostic procedure in which a catheter is inserted into an artery at the groin or arm and pushed through to the heart. A dye is injected through this catheter into the arteries and chambers of the heart while an X-ray camera takes a series of pictures. The procedure can clearly show blocked areas where the dye cannot flow. Dr. Hirschfeld explained that it is a relatively painless, highly sophisticated procedure, which must be performed by specialists at major medical centers. When he asked where I would like to have it done, I named the Cleveland Clinic, about one hundred miles from Findlay. Dr. Hirschfeld called the Clinic and requested an appointment for me. Because of the number of cases seen at the Clinic, the first available appointment would be six weeks away, in February.

"In the meantime," the doctor advised me, "don't do anything too strenuous and try to avoid emotional stress." He gave me a prescription for nitroglycerin to take when angina pains occurred, and he advised me to avoid foods that are high in cholesterol and saturated fats.

I walked out of the doctor's office in a daze. I couldn't believe it: I had heart disease! How was this possible? I had always been the picture of health. I was still a young man, vigorous and strong, and I felt fine. The angina pain seemed almost trifling to me, certainly nothing to disable me or to interfere with my activities. I wanted to believe that somehow the test had been wrong, but I knew, deep down, that it wasn't.

I drove to the pharmacy still in a daze, picked up my prescription, and drove home. I still couldn't accept the reality of what I had just learned, even though I tried to comprehend how I had changed from a person who had been "in excellent health" in my annual physical examination a few weeks earlier. I kept my New Year's Eve date and joined my friends for dinner and a large cocktail party. If I seemed particularly withdrawn or preoccupied that evening, none of my friends remarked about it.

When I returned to work the day after New Year's, the pressure was still on. Marathon's management had decided that the only viable way to avoid the Mobil takeover was to enter a friendly merger agreement with a "white knight" company, in this case, U.S. Steel Corporation. They were fighting Mobil in the courts to gain time for U.S. Steel's merger offer to be effected. On January 6, my boss informed me that we had another crucial publication deadline to meet. My staff and I had to write and publish another special edition of an employee publication the next day because it was crucial to

1. A Case of Heart Disease

keep the employees up to date on the latest developments in the takeover fight.

I went home after work and began planning writing assignments, photography assignments, and the layout work we would need to do on extremely short notice. It would require another eighteen- to twenty-hour effort by the staff and myself under great pressure to meet the deadline. I don't recall what I ate for dinner. Afterward, I sat on a sofa and watched television, trying to forget the anxiety I felt about the project ahead of me at work.

Suddenly I began having angina pain. I was surprised to have it occur when I wasn't exercising; I had believed angina was only triggered by exertion. A nitroglycerin tablet under the tongue relieved the pain, but a half hour later it struck again. I repeated the nitroglycerin dose, but in another half hour the pain was back. This isn't right, I thought. Finally, at ten o'clock, I called Dr. Hirschfeld's number. He was out of town, but the answering service put me in touch with the doctor on duty for the group, Jerome Beekman, a cardiologist. When I described my symptoms, he said it sounded like unstable angina, a type that is not brought on by exertion. When I told him I lived alone, he didn't like my situation and advised me to come to the hospital immediately, where I could be monitored and attended to. I threw a bathrobe and my shaving kit into an overnight bag and called a taxi to take me to the hospital, only a mile away. Then I called my ex-wife in Pennsylvania so that somebody in my family would know where I was going; I asked her to call my children, who lived in Connecticut, Illinois, and Colorado. It was a lonely and worrisome trip to the hospital, but I was anxious to get to a place where I could have medical attention.

Findlay's Blanchard Valley Hospital is, in my opinion, an exceptionally fine small-city hospital, and it has an up-to-date coronary care unit. I was quickly admitted to this unit, where Dr. Beekman visited me within a half hour of my arrival. I was hooked up to a heart monitor. At first it was comforting to know I was getting medical attention, but not long afterward I began having a series of angina attacks that lasted through the night. As I lay there, wondering what was happening to me, the possibility of death struck me for the first time in my life. I wondered if I would die of a heart attack before morning. I thought about my family and how my death would affect them, and I wondered about all the unfinished projects in my life, such as a book I was writing for a publisher in the East. Then, absurdly, I worried about how my office staff was going to cope with the rush project. Surprisingly, the possibility of death didn't terrify me, as I had always thought it would. I've had a good life, I thought, and if it has to end now, so be it.

But morning came and I was still there. Dr. Beekman and the staff on duty, however, were concerned that they hadn't been able to eliminate my unstable angina with medication. "I believe you're flirting with a heart attack," Dr. Beekman told me. "I've talked with Dr. Hirschfeld about it, and we believe you should have a catheterization exam as quickly as possible to see if

1. A Case of Heart Disease

coronary bypass surgery is indicated." Dr. Hirschfeld called the Cleveland Clinic that morning and arranged for an emergency-priority appointment for cardiac catheterization the next day. By now, my angina attacks had ceased and my condition seemed to stabilize as the day went on. It was decided that I should make the two-hour trip to Cleveland by ambulance, with a registered nurse in attendance. The trip was pleasant and comfortable. My spirits were lifted with the knowledge that I was going to receive some of the best medical care in the world, and I chatted with the friendly, personable nurse during the trip.

Arriving at the Cleveland Clinic is an impressive experience, whether you do so by ambulance or in your own car. It is an enormous complex of buildings in a campus setting on Cleveland's crowded east side. The buildings seem to be always increasing in number, as one expansion program follows another. But the Clinic's contributions to medicine and its worldwide reputation are even more impressive. As the second largest group medical practice in the world, the Clinic has a long list of major accomplishments in many areas of medicine, including advancements in the treatment of cancer, kidney disease, brain and nervous system disorders, and urogenital and reproductive disorders. The development of artificial organs and joints is another important research area. But the Clinic's reputation for advancements in the treatment of cardiovascular disease was what I was familiar with. It was here that left cardiac catheterization and selective coronary arteriography were devel-

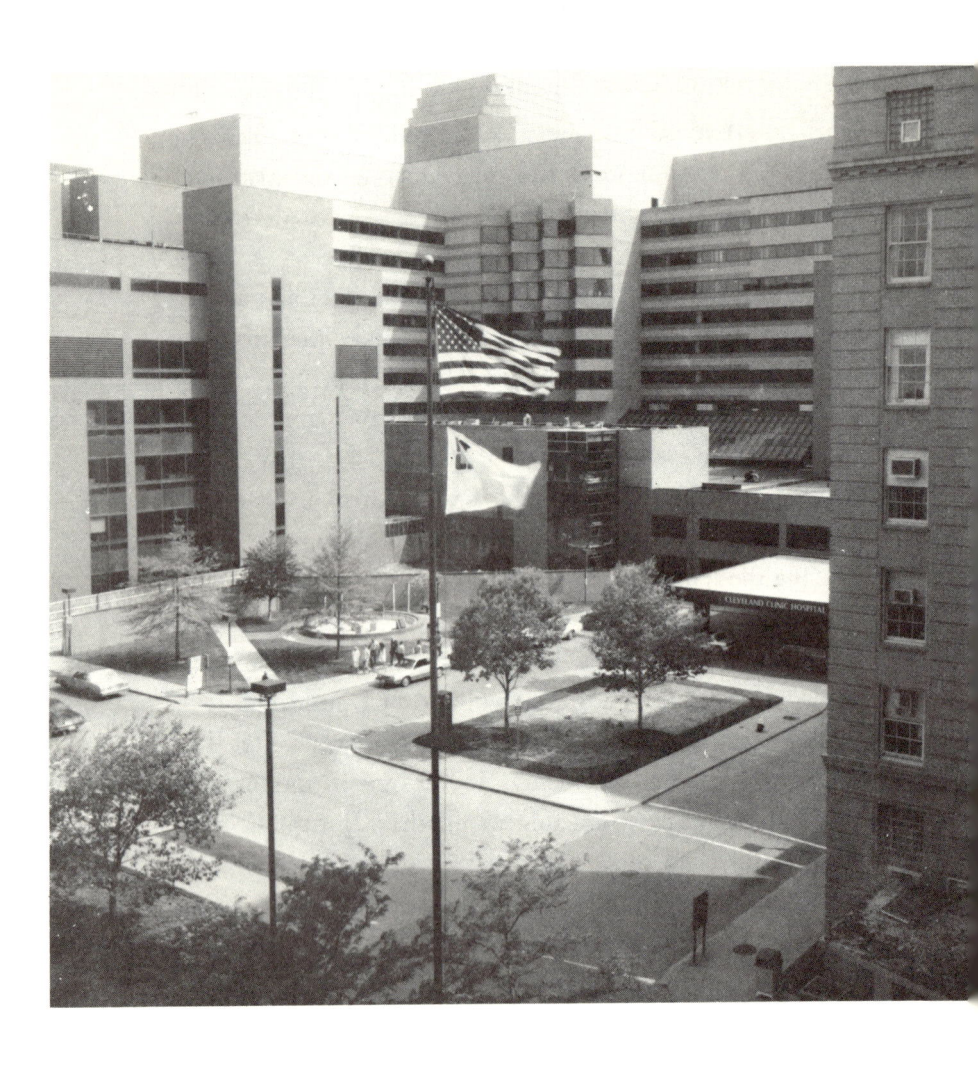

The main entrance to the Cleveland Clinic Foundation's collection of buildings and facilities. It was here that cardiac catheterization and the pinpointing of coronary artery blockage through X-ray movies (angiograms) was developed, making coronary bypass surgery possible. The first successful saphenous vein bypass operation was performed here in 1967, ushering in the era of coronary bypass surgery.

1. A Case of Heart Disease

oped by Dr. F. Mason Sones, Jr., in 1958, providing the first—and still the best—means of accurately pinpointing coronary artery blockage and other heart defects. Without it, there would be no coronary bypass surgery today. And it was also here, in 1967, that Dr. Rene Favaloro performed the first successful saphenous vein bypass operation on a patient with a blocked artery. Since then, the Cleveland Clinic has had more clinical experience with this operation than any other medical center in the world. More than 32,000 patients have had bypass surgery here in the past dozen years. The King of Saudi Arabia, the president of Brazil, and a number of other celebrities came here for bypass operations. Many other medical centers do wonderful work with bypass surgery, too, but the Cleveland Clinic is called "The Mecca" by many physicians. They're not just surgeons here, though; the Clinic's cardiology group is also famous for their expertise and advances in the diagnosis and nonsurgical treatment of heart disease.

My case was referred to Dr. Earl Shirey of the cardiology staff. As I was admitted to my room, I asked a nurse about Dr. Shirey. "He's one of the most distinguished cardiologists in medicine," she said. "He's been on the staff since 1957 and he assisted Dr. Sones when he developed coronary arteriography, back in 1958." I was elated—how could I do better than that in the choice of a doctor to perform my cardiac catheterization? It pays to come to The Mecca, I thought.

The next morning, Dr. Shirey met with me and explained the catheterization procedure. His warm, friendly manner, innate courtesy, and wealth of knowledge put me completely at ease, and I wasn't the least bit nervous as I was wheeled into the catheterization laboratory. This is not to say that heart catheterization should be taken lightly; it is an invasive procedure that carries a slight risk of injury or death, depending on the individual. However, when the procedure is performed by a highly experienced physician, the risk is very low.

My catheterization was routine and painless. I was given a local anesthetic in the crook of my right arm while strapped to a table that could be tilted and turned. The table was surrounded by an X-ray camera and other equipment that record information on the patient's condition. An electrocardiograph was also hooked up to monitor heart function. I didn't feel much of anything as Dr. Shirey inserted the catheter into my arm, nor did I feel anything as he worked it up my arm and into my heart. An X-ray television monitor was positioned so that I could watch it along with Dr. Shirey. I could see the line of the catheter as it entered my heart—a fascinating sight. "Now you're going to feel a hot, flushed sensation as I release the dye into your bloodstream," Dr. Shirey warned. Indeed, I did feel an intense hot flush for a moment, but it was not painful. I could see the dye flowing on the X-ray monitor. In a few moments, the test was over and the catheter was withdrawn. The small incision in my arm was stitched up painlessly under local anesthetic; then I was taken back to my room.

A few hours later, I met with Dr. Shirey to discuss the findings of the examination. It showed what other

1. A Case of Heart Disease

medical tests could not show: I had a definite blockage in my coronary arteries. "Your right artery has some minor narrowing in places, but not enough to impede blood flow significantly," he said. "Now, as you probably have heard, the left main artery is the one that is most crucial to the heart's functioning. If the left main trunk is blocked significantly, it is usually dangerous and life-threatening. Your left main trunk has some mild, diffuse irregularity in the pattern of blood flow, but not enough to cause us immediate concern. However, the anterior descending left artery, beginning where it branches from the main trunk, is totally obstructed. This is a very important artery because it feeds oxygen to a large part of the heart. The middle and distal segments of this anterior descending artery are being supplied with some blood from the right coronary artery through what we call collaterals: small vessels that grow toward the blocked artery to substitute blood supply. You also have blockage of 40 to 50 percent in two places in your left circumflex artery, which carries blood laterally across the heart, as you can see on this chart. In addition, there is some blockage of smaller branches of the circumflex."

My first question was whether or not I would need to have coronary bypass surgery. "You have what is classified medically as severe double vessel coronary heart disease, and that makes you a candidate for bypass surgery, but it doesn't mean that surgery is mandatory," Dr. Shirey explained.

I had heard in conversations with fellow workers that

big medical-center physicians were quick to recommend bypass surgery, rather than conservative treatment with medication, but this certainly wasn't true here. Dr. Shirey explained that such medication as beta blockers and calcium channel blockers, along with others, could lessen the frequency and severity of angina attacks if I chose not to have surgery. He went on to point out that diet, exercise, and lack of stress could all help me to live reasonably comfortably with my arterial blockages. The blockages would still be obstructing blood supply, but with proper medication and attention to life-style factors, the effect wouldn't be as great. He asked me to think it over, talk with my family, or with other doctors if I wished, and then make my decision.

That evening in my room I discussed it with my ex-wife who had come from Pennsylvania to visit me. I also talked with my children by telephone, but I had already made my decision and I just wanted my family's reaction. My tendency has always been to say, "If something is wrong, fix it," no matter what the problem. I didn't agonize over this decision because to me it was just something else wrong that needed to be fixed. Dr. Shirey had pointed out that if the bypass operation was successful, I could probably return to a normal life and be free from angina pains. "It's not a cure for heart disease, but it's a palliative that can make your life better for a while," he said.

That sounded better to me than the conservative medication approach. Having recently faced my own mortality for the first time, I understood more clearly than

1. A Case of Heart Disease

ever before that I didn't know how much time I had left to live. And I decided that I would rather live that allotted time feeling fit and free of angina, if that was what bypass surgery could do for me. Of course, there was no guarantee that the operation would produce those results. There is some risk of death in any open heart surgery, for one thing. But I knew the mortality rate for bypass surgery at the Cleveland Clinic was among the lowest in the world—less than 1 percent. I also knew that not all bypass operations were successful in supplying the heart with more blood and freeing the patient from angina. But most of them were successful, and I knew the odds were in my favor.

The next morning, I met with Dr. Shirey again and told him of my decision. I asked if there was any way I could schedule the operation immediately, since I was already at the Cleveland Clinic. To my surprise, he managed to schedule my operation for the next day. I had dreaded the thought of going home and waiting a month or more for the surgery. I wanted to get it over with, while I was in an optimistic frame of mind, rather than brood about all that could go wrong while I waited.

During the rest of that day and evening, I received telephone calls from relatives and old friends from Massachusetts, Washington, Florida, California, and other parts of the country. My ex-wife had called many of them and told them of my illness, and they responded with such an outpouring of calls and good wishes that I hardly had time to worry. I remember talking and laughing with my sister in Massachusetts while I was being shaved for the next day's surgery. I'm sure the medication given me included some sort of tranquilizer, because I was relaxed all evening.

I was awakened by a nurse the next morning, having slept soundly, thanks to a sleeping pill. I shaved and brushed my teeth, finishing just as my ex-wife arrived. I felt nervous about what was going to happen, but it was not a strong fear of death. We chatted about inconsequential things as relatives usually do in hospital rooms. I kept thinking about the possibility that I might not come out of the operating room alive. But I felt so secure to be in the hands of the Cleveland Clinic's surgical team that I doubted I would die.

Soon two hospital attendants came into the room with a bed on wheels. I slid onto it from my bed and was covered with a sheet. The attendants began to push the bed cart out the door. I managed a faint smile to my ex-wife, who said she'd be waiting to see me in the intensive care room as soon as they allowed her in. I wondered if I would see her or anyone else again. But it was too late to be terror-stricken, and I accepted the fact that I had no power to decide my fate now. The mild medication I had been given a short time earlier helped, of course, to keep me calm and as relaxed as possible, under the circumstances.

It seemed like a long ride through the corridors, my only view being the overhead lights. In a few minutes I arrived at the preparation area, or induction room. Medical personnel attached some wire leads to various parts of my body. These leads would be hooked up to monitoring

1. A Case of Heart Disease

equipment so the doctors and staff could keep track of my body functions during the operation. My hospital gown was removed and I lay naked under the sheet.

A short time later, I was wheeled into the operating room, which was smaller than I had imagined it would be. The room was crammed with machinery and monitoring devices, attended to by several nurses and technicians. I remember shivering in my unclothed state because it was very chilly in the room; the air-conditioning was going full blast. I later learned that operating rooms are kept at these chilly temperatures to counteract the heat from the high-intensity lights and to retard the growth of germs. Two young resident surgeons introduced themselves; they would be assisting Dr. Delos Cosgrove, the surgeon in charge of the operation. I was in a fairly drowsy state but generally aware of what was going on as the surgical team members busied themselves preparing for the operation. Next, Dr. Cosgrove came into the room briefly and introduced himself to me. That's the last I remember of the operating room. The anesthesiologist released his magic potion and put me to sleep swiftly.

An instant later, it seemed to me, I faintly heard a nurse saying, "Wake up, Norman. The operation is over." I had the sensation that I was at the bottom of a deep well and that someone was calling down to me from above. I was in such a deep sleep that I didn't seem to be able to rouse myself. The nurse repeated insistently, "Wake up, Norman. The operation is over!" I remember thinking that I must be dead or dying, and it was futile to try to revive me. But after a few minutes, I did wake, feeling very groggy. Wires and catheters seemed to be sticking into me everywhere, and an oxygen tube was in my throat. I was uncomfortable and aching, but the pain wasn't excruciating. The attractive nurse who hovered over me truly seemed to be my angel of mercy. I felt she was the one person in the world who would help me live and get better.

I was in the intensive care, or recovery room. There were no windows, and the walls were lined with beds occupied by about a dozen other patients. As I looked around, bleary-eyed, in the dim lights, the place seemed like Dante's Inferno or maybe a scene from a science fiction movie, since all my fellow sufferers had tubes and wires protruding from them. I don't remember much about the rest of my stay in the recovery room, which I believe lasted twenty-four hours. The morphine and any other pain-killing medicines kept me in a sort of dreamlike state. Eventually a nurse removed the catheters and wires from my body and took me in a wheelchair to a regular room. The nurses at the Cleveland Clinic must be among the best in the world—astute, compassionate, knowledgeable, and cheerful. I never met a grouchy, officious, or uncaring nurse there during my entire stay. Their role is absolutely vital to the well-being and recuperation of any patient, and they perform it admirably.

During my first couple of days back in a regular hospital room, I remained giddy and on a sort of "high" from the medication. But I had to endure the aching chest and leg, from which my saphenous vein was re-

1. A Case of Heart Disease

moved, and I was definitely uncomfortable. Like all patients, I was instructed to exercise my lungs to clear the fluid that can collect in them. I was given a plastic toy-like device and told to inhale through its mouth tube. This caused a ping-pong ball in a vertical tube to rise. It would fall back to the bottom when I ran out of breath. At frequent intervals throughout the day, I was encouraged to thus exercise my lungs several times in succession. I was also told to cough frequently to loosen the phlegm in my lungs. With a breastbone and ribs that had been split open and then wired together, it was very painful to cough. The nurses told me to hold a pillow against my chest when I coughed, to ease the pain.

On the second day in my room, I was able to get up and go to the bathroom, and soon I was able to take showers. I had a fleeting, irrational fear that the stream from the shower would split my chest incision open the first time I tried it, but the water felt wonderful. Showering and shaving wore me out the first few times I tried them, and I had to take a nap immediately afterward. Also on the second day, I was encouraged to walk out of my room and down the hall to the nursing station. A nurse told me that one complete walk down the hall, around the nursing station and the central area, then back, was one-tenth of a mile. She told me not to overdo it at first, but that I should try to reach a goal of ten trips as soon as I could. I felt weak and wobbly the first few times I walked this circuit, and I had to lie down and rest after each trip. But this weakness quickly passed, and I reached my goal of a mile on my second day. After several days, I was walking up to two miles a day.

Walking was, in fact, high on the list of recommendations for my convalescence period at home. To help educate patients about their recuperation, a special "class" is held in the hospital a few days before discharge. More than a dozen of us gathered in a room furnished like a school classroom, with a chalkboard, a lectern, and rows of folding chairs for the "students." A young woman who was either a nurse or a medical technician conducted the class, explaining that it was important for us to know the things we should do to help us recuperate as quickly as possible so we could resume our normal lives. We should begin by walking two miles a day if possible, and then gradually increase this distance if we wished. We should wait at least three weeks before driving a car. Flying in a commercial airliner posed no risks if we had to travel a great distance home. We should continue the breathing exercises with the plastic device, and we should wear an elastic surgical stocking to reduce the swelling in the leg from which the saphenous veins had been removed. The class lasted about an hour, and most of the patients took notes and asked questions.

Dr. Shirey visited me on his rounds. He was pleased with my progress, and his cheerfulness and optimism were contagious. His encouragement soon had me thinking about the unrestricted, pain-free life I could have ahead of me once I had fully recovered. My mood was upbeat most of the time, with none of the depression

1. A Case of Heart Disease 25

that I'd heard was common for postoperative heart patients. I credit Dr. Shirey and the cheerful nurses for this.

I was also visited by Dr. Robert Adams, one of the physicians who assisted Dr. Cosgrove with my surgery. He showed me a diagram of a heart and told me about the operation. The obstruction in my left anterior descending artery was bypassed by grafting one end of my left internal mammary artery, which runs inside the chest wall, to a place below the obstruction. Thus blood would be able to flow from this chest artery directly into my coronary artery. He explained that surgeons favor using the left internal mammary artery if possible because experience has shown that it tends to remain unclogged longer than the saphenous leg veins. Of course, there are only two of these arteries, a left and a right, so operations with multiple bypass grafts require the leg veins as well. Six or seven years seems to be an average length of time for saphenous vein grafts to remain unclogged, whereas mammary artery grafts commonly remain open for a decade or longer.

A segment of the saphenous vein from my left leg had been grafted between my aorta and my partially blocked left circumflex artery, bypassing the obstruction. The operation was routine, with no difficulties, Dr. Adams told me.

Six days after my operation I was discharged. My ex-wife drove me to Findlay, then returned to her job in Pennsylvania. So that I did not have to spend my first two weeks at home alone, my daughter, Gayle, took vacation time from her job in Boulder, Colorado and spent them with me. She was waiting when I arrived at home, as was my son, Greg, who had driven from his Chicago home for a two-day visit. I was still taking Darvocet tablets for my chest and leg pain, and I still napped once or twice a day, but I was gaining strength daily. Gayle accompanied me on my walks every day, which sometimes took place at a nearby shopping mall because of the January weather. Sometimes I walked in circles at home, from the kitchen through a hallway, the living room, the dining room, and back to the kitchen. I didn't mind the exercise much, but boredom was a problem. I couldn't watch television while walking in circles at home, and even the various sights at the shopping mall wore thin after a few days. On days when the weather was better, we walked around Findlay, which was more enjoyable.

I had a routine recovery at home, with no particular problems. The pain faded fairly soon and I didn't feel bad at all. But I had been advised not to go back to my job for about eight weeks. Meanwhile, the high stress on the job looked as if it could be reduced in the near future, because Marathon won its fight against Mobil. The merger agreement with U.S. Steel was accompanied by an announcement that there were no plans to move Marathon's headquarters out of Findlay, or to eliminate anybody's job. The people of Findlay gave a tremendous sigh, relieved that their nice little city was spared the economic catastrophe of having Marathon's headquarters close. The employees of Marathon were overjoyed, too,

1. A Case of Heart Disease

that their jobs were spared, and business soon returned to normal at the office.

I drove back to the Cleveland Clinic by myself for my six-week checkup with Dr. Shirey. I told him that I had not experienced any angina since my operation and that, generally, I was feeling fine. I was also given advice by Dr. Shirey on how to maintain my pain-free condition and good cardiovascular functioning. In addition to advising me to avoid foods high in cholesterol and animal fats, he encouraged me to continue my daily walking and other exercise. "We in medicine don't have as much knowledge as we would like about the effects of exercise on heart disease," he said, "but the right kind of exercise can't hurt you and it may help to prolong your angina-free status. Besides, exercise has other benefits: it helps you reduce and control your weight. And weight reduction often helps lower serum cholesterol and triglycerides as well as high blood pressure. We're still learning more about the effects of emotional stress on heart disease, too, but there's enough experience for us to know that it is a risk factor. If you have a high-stress job or situation in your personal life, you should try to take steps to reduce this stress." He advised me to continue taking the 10-milligram Isordil tablets that I had been taking with each meal and at bedtime. Isordil is a nitrate that dilates the coronary arteries, to increase blood flow to the heart.

Since that six-week checkup in March 1982, I have returned to the Cleveland Clinic each year for my annual company physical. On each occasion, I have also scheduled an appointment with Dr. Shirey and undergone a thallium stress test. This is the usual treadmill stress test with an electrocardiograph, but it has an added diagnostic procedure. When the patient's heart rate is highest on the treadmill, a low-grade radioactive agent or "dye" is injected into the bloodstream through a catheter. When the treadmill exercise is finished, the patient spends two thirty-minute periods in a series of prone positions, being photographed by a special camera that shows the flow of the dye through the coronary arteries and the heart chambers. The films show how much blood (and oxygen) is entering the heart. A recurrence of coronary artery obstructions would diminish the flow of blood to the heart. As of this writing, the findings on my thallium stress tests have been negative, indicating a satisfactory blood flow. I find it reassuring to take this test each year. There have been some changes on my electrocardiograms in the years since my bypass surgery, but I understand it is quite common to see changes after such surgery. I might worry more about these changes were it not for the reassurance of the negative thallium stress test each year.

It's easy to become something of a hypochondriac when you have heart disease. And make no mistake about it, you *do* have heart disease even after you have coronary bypass surgery. The surgery can free you from angina and make you feel healthy again, as though you had been given a "fresh start," but as Dr. Shirey cautioned me, "You still have heart disease. The underlying disease is still there, gradually clogging your arteries

1. A Case of Heart Disease

and even the new bypass grafts. There is no way of knowing how long you'll go without having problems again because of insufficient blood supply to your heart."

From time to time I have had chest pains, and they sometimes worry me. Once I even was admitted to the hospital in Findlay so that my enzyme levels, heart rate, and other signs could be monitored to see if I were having severe heart trouble. The findings were negative, as they have been each time I have complained of chest pains. Cardiac trouble has been eliminated as a cause each time, and the consensus has been that the pains are in my chest wall and are caused by something other than my heart (there are many causes of chest pains besides an ailing heart). I have been reassured each time I have had such pains and found they were not caused by cardiac trouble, and by paying attention to them, have gradually learned to differentiate them from angina. I have not had any episodes resembling the pain of the angina I remember from the period before my bypass surgery. For a while I thought I was a hypochondriac, but doctors have repeatedly advised me not to ignore chest pains unless I can recognize them as muscle or some other type of pain. Now that I have learned to recognize different types of pains from experience, I'm less likely to panic and wonder if the pain is angina or a heart attack. If I were to experience an unfamiliar pain or other symptoms that worried me, I would check it out with a physician as soon as possible, but that hasn't happened for a couple of years.

Heart disease forces anyone to come to terms with his

or her own mortality. I don't know how much longer I have to live, but then none of us does, heart disease or not. I think about my father, who lived an active life despite his angina for more than thirty years, even though he ate foods high in fat and cholesterol and smoked. Then I read in the papers about young men dying of heart attacks with no symptoms. Heart disease is such a difficult affliction to understand that even the best minds in medical science can't predict its course accurately. There is enough evidence of the effects of such risk factors as smoking, high blood pressure, diets high in cholesterol and saturated fats, stress, and lack of exercise to indicate that most of us can avoid heart disease and live longer if we cut down on or eliminate those factors. But there is no way to tell accurately how long an individual can avoid heart disease or how long he or she will live.

Despite this uncertainty, I'm glad I chose to have coronary bypass surgery. It has already given me several years of pain-free, unrestricted life, which I am enjoying to the fullest. I have traveled internationally, written books, and performed my job with vigor and enthusiasm since my operation. I play tennis, swim, sail, hike, ski cross-country, and enjoy a very active social life. I have found warmth, emotional security, and romantic love with a wonderful woman in Ohio. Emotional stress has been reduced in my life, and I have tried to reduce my other risk factors, too. I eat virtually no red meat these days, no eggs, whole milk, or other foods high in cholesterol. I have not had as much success in avoiding baked

1. A Case of Heart Disease

desserts and controlling my sweet tooth. But I do get regular exercise on a motorized treadmill in my home, and I have stopped smoking my pipe. These are really small sacrifices to make in return for better odds for a healthy life.

It is incumbent on those of us with heart disease to learn as much about it as possible, rather than fear the unknown. That is the purpose of this book.

2.
Nature's Marvelous Pump

THE HUMAN HEART has always been viewed with awe and has had magical powers ascribed to it. In medieval times, it was regarded as the noblest organ in the body, the very core of a human being. In popular usage, the heart has represented courage ("take heart"), the center of things ("the heart of the matter"), and the source of romantic emotions (thousands of poems and songs with the word *heart* in them, heart-shaped valentines, and so on). These ideas were formed before medical science had much realistic knowledge of the heart. Yet today, when so much is known about the anatomy and physiology of the heart, the awe and wonder with which the heart is regarded remain intense.

Now we understand that it is essentially a pump. But it is the most marvelous pump ever seen. Consider this: It weighs less than a pound and is generally no larger than a grapefruit, yet it pumps about ten pints of blood a minute through some 60,000 miles of blood vessels.

2. Nature's Marvelous Pump

The heart beats about 100,000 times a day; and it goes on to beat some 2.5 billion times in an average lifetime, pumping enough blood in that time to fill a football stadium.

In an average adult, the heart beats (contracts) about sixty to eighty times a minute when the body is at rest. The rate goes up by 20 to 30 percent when we walk, because more blood must be circulated as the body uses more energy, and it goes up even further with more exertion, up to the maximum rate, which is normally about 200 beats a minute for a 25-year-old. The maximum rate declines with age. Exercise can improve the efficiency of the body's circulatory system so the heart doesn't have to work as hard to pump blood through the body. This is why the heart, or pulse, rate of well-conditioned athletes is usually much lower than that of other people.

The volume of blood pumped by the heart is about the same for each beat, whatever the pulse rate. A beat is actually a contraction of the heart muscle, much like the clenching of a fist, and each contraction usually squeezes about two and one-half ounces of blood out of the heart to the blood vessels.

Compared to the functioning of the brain, the heart goes about its work with wonderful simplicity. The organ is divided into four chambers, two on top and two on the bottom. Each upper chamber is known as an atrium, the lower chambers as ventricles. The upper chambers, or atria, receive blood from veins and serve as reservoirs.

The atria send this blood into the ventricles below. The ventricles are the pumping chambers of the heart, and each ventricle does a different job. The left ventricle pumps blood to all the parts of the body except the lungs. That is the job of the right ventricle. The two chambers are separated by a wall of muscle about half-an-inch thick, the septum.

The blood goes from one chamber to another and out of the heart through four valves, which act like one-way doors, letting blood flow through them in only one direction. Each valve has two or three flaps, the leaflets or cusps, which open and close with the force of the blood in the heart. The two valves (the inlet valves) between the atria and the ventricles below are the mitral valve and the tricuspid valve. The two valves that open to let blood flow out of the heart and into the aorta and the pulmonary artery, respectively, are called the aortic valve and the pulmonary valve; they are outlet valves.

Here's how they work: As the atria fill with blood, the pressure above the valves is greater than the pressure below them. The atria contract, and the pressure of the blood forces the inlet valves open, which allow the blood to flow freely into the ventricles. Then as the ventricles fill with blood, they also contract. When this happens, the valves snap shut and stop blood from flowing backward, up to the atria. At the same time, the two outlet valves, the aortic and the pulmonary, open because of the higher pressure in the filled ventricles. Blood moves through them into the aorta and the pulmonary artery.

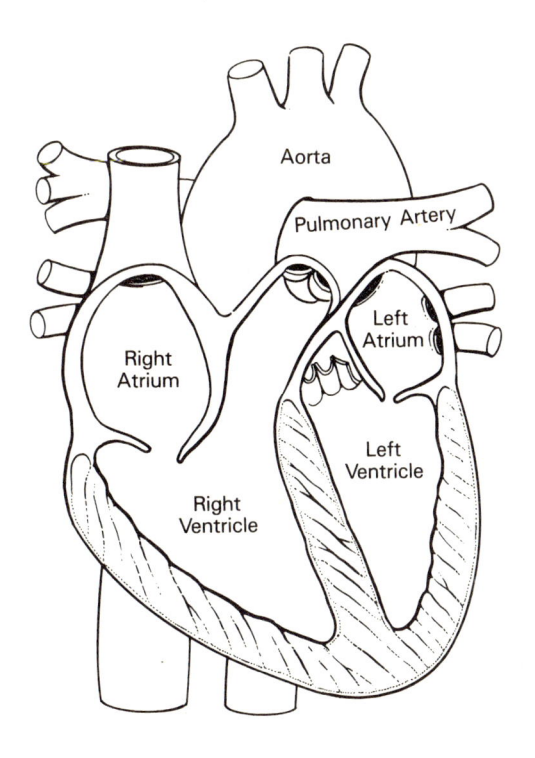

The heart, nature's marvelous pump, is divided into four chambers. The two upper chambers, the right and left atria, receive the blood that has circulated throughout the body and serve as reservoirs. When they contract, the pressure forces blood through valves into the ventricles below them. The ventricles are the pumping chambers, each with a different job to do. The right ventricle pumps blood through a valve to the pulmonary artery, which carries it to the lungs, where carbon dioxide is discharged and oxygen is restored to it. The oxygen-rich blood then travels to the left atrium, where it is forced through a valve into the left ventricle. This ventricle pumps the blood vigorously through another valve into the aorta, which carries the blood into other vessels for distribution throughout the body. The entire circulatory system is amazingly efficient; the heart typically pumps about 10 pints of blood per minute through some 60,000 miles of blood vessels in the body. It beats about 100,000 times a day.

The "heartbeat" sound that can be heard through a stethoscope is produced by the closing of the valves. Doctors usually describe these sounds as lub-dub, a pause, lub-dub, a pause, and so on. The "lub," or first sound, is made partly by the closing of the mitral and tricuspid valves. The "dub," or second sound, is made by the closing of the aortic and pulmonary valves.

The entire circulatory system, including the heart and lungs, is amazingly efficient. Every organ and tissue of the body requires oxygen and other nutrients to function. The network of vessels that make up this system is more complex than any manmade network of pipes. The freshly oxygenated blood is pumped out of the heart through the largest artery, the aorta, which is about one inch in diameter, and then through progressively smaller vessels. The blood vessels branch out into the tiny arterioles, and then to even tinier vessels—the capillaries, which are so tiny that they can only be seen through a microscope. There are ten billion capillaries, which are so narrow that red blood cells must pass through them single file. It is here that the oxygen and nutrients carried by the blood are delivered to the tissues and organs. Then the blood picks up carbon dioxide and cell wastes for disposal and starts its return journey to the heart. The blood moves from the capillaries into bigger vessels called venules, then to the large vessels, the veins, which go back to the right atrium through the body's largest veins, the vena cavae. The blood moves from the right atrium through the tricuspid valve into the right ventricle. There it is pumped through the pulmonary

2. Nature's Marvelous Pump

valve and pulmonary artery to the lungs, where carbon dioxide is released and oxygen is taken up. It then begins the next cycle, bringing oxygen-rich blood back to the left atrium and then the left ventricle, ready to be pumped throughout the body.

Curiously enough, the pump for all this blood needs a vascular system of its own to receive blood, like any other part of the body. Though the heart is constantly flooded with blood, its thick walls, with their liquid-tight lining, prevent it from taking nourishment from the blood within it. Instead the heart muscle has its own network of large and small blood vessels to supply it with nutrients and oxygen. The largest vessels in this network are the coronary arteries. The name comes from the Latin word for *crown*, because they encircle the heart on the outside surface somewhat like a crown.

The two main coronary arteries, the left and the right, branch off from the aorta. They are the first branches to receive the blood as it moves through the aorta on its way to other parts of the body. The left main coronary artery divides into two slightly smaller arteries: the left anterior descending, which runs diagonally down the front of the heart, and the left circumflex, which circles laterally around to the back of the heart. These are very important arteries; they bring most of the blood to the left side of the heart. The right side of the heart is supplied with blood by the right coronary artery. The coronary arteries are only one-fourth of an inch in diameter at their widest, and they branch into smaller and smaller vessels.

Nature has a way of trying to make up for deficiencies in the blood supply to the heart. In many cases, if one of the large coronary arteries becomes narrowed or blocked, as a result of coronary artery disease, the smaller vessels grow wider and longer and sometimes join small branches of another artery to help compensate for the diminished blood supply caused by the blockage.

The system responsible for this pumping and circulation of blood must not stop, or the person will quickly die. The heart must coordinate the contractions of the atria and the ventricles to correspond with the opening and closing of the heart's valves. To regulate this sequence, the heart has a natural electrical conduction system. The system is triggered by a tiny bundle of cells, the sinoatrial (SA) node, at the top of the right atrium. Electrical signals from the SA node set the split-second pace for the heartbeat. The electrical current is conducted through the heart in a pathway of muscle fibers that leads to another node, the atrioventricular (AV) node in the heart's center. The electrical current moves from the atria down to the ventricles, and stimulates them, in turn, to contract. This is what makes the heart contract and relax rhythmically. It is a precision operation—the average heartbeat lasts from 0.15 to 0.3 second—and it can go on for one hundred years or more. We have yet to see an engineering feat that matches this wonderful system.

3.
Heart Disease: What Goes Wrong with the Pump

As with a manmade mechanical pump and piping system, a number of things can go wrong with the human heart and cause the heart to malfunction. Unfortunately, things go wrong in such a great number of people that cardiovascular disease, in its variety of forms, is by far the leading cause of death in the United States. The American Heart Association's figures for one recent year, 1983, showed that more than 63 million Americans have one form or more of heart or blood vessel disease. Some 57 million of these have high blood pressure (hypertension). About 4.7 million people have diagnosed cases of coronary heart disease, and 2 million have rheumatic heart disease. Stroke victims number almost 2 million.

The number of deaths from cardiovascular disease in 1983 totaled 989,400, which represents nearly one-half of all deaths. This compares with 440,620 for cancer and 91,290 for accidents. And if we look at only one category of cardiovascular disease deaths in that year—heart attacks—the figure of 547,100 is still higher than that for any other cause of death.

Easily the most common form of cardiac disorder in the United States is coronary artery disease. Although a number of diseases can affect the vital coronary arteries, in about 99 percent of the cases, the problem is atherosclerosis. It's easy to confuse this name with the general term arteriosclerosis, popularly known as "hardening of the arteries." But atherosclerosis is a certain kind of arteriosclerosis in which the lining of the arteries is thickened and roughened by soft fatty deposits, called atheromas. As they thicken, the arteries become less flexible and progressively narrower inside as the deposits build up and harden.

Eventually this process can completely obstruct an artery, but even before that happens, the deposits can cause blood to form a clot at the site of the narrowing. Normally, blood cells do not stick to artery walls, but certain kinds of blood cells, the platelets, pile up and die on the fatty atheromas. Tiny, threadlike structures, fibrils, form on the dead platelets. The matted fibrils and the platelets mesh to form a hard solidly massed blood clot. The clot may grow larger until it eventually obstructs the artery. Sometimes the clot breaks loose and is carried through the body's network of vessels until it obstructs a narrower vessel somewhere else in the body.

Medical science still does not have unassailable knowledge of the causes of atherosclerosis, but a great many dedicated scientists throughout the world have spent

3. Heart Disease

many years conducting thousands of studies and experiments to learn more about it. They have compiled a growing body of knowledge that, though it is not absolute proof, strongly suggests that there are a number of factors, individually and in combination, that probably have important roles in causing this disease. Many years of experience and study have identified such risk factors as smoking, hypertension, obesity, family history, high cholesterol levels, and diabetes. These risk factors will be discussed in Chapter Four.

When atherosclerosis produces a narrowing of a coronary artery, the blood supply to the heart muscle is reduced. When a muscle or tissue of the body does not receive enough blood (and hence, oxygen) the condition is called ischemia, and when this occurs in the heart, or one area of the heart, it often produces a symptom called angina. Millions of people with heart disease are familiar with the pain of angina. Although the pain may differ from one person to another, the most common experiences are to feel it as a dull, crushing pain in the middle of the chest, which sometimes spreads to the upper arms, the neck, or the jaw.

However, angina takes more than one form. Stable angina is usually brought on by physical exertion: running, climbing stairs, shoveling snow, or even walking. Anything that requires the heart to pump more quickly causes it to need more oxygen, and if an obstruction in the coronary arteries prevents the extra blood and oxygen from getting to the heart when it needs it, the heart "complains" through angina pain. Most stable angina lasts less than ten minutes and ceases when the activity is halted or after the drug nitroglycerin is taken. Nitroglycerin (and some other drugs) dilate the blood vessels, allowing more blood to pass to the heart muscle. People who have experienced stable angina pains usually learn to expect them when they engage in certain activities. Stable angina can be quite predictable.

Unstable angina is another story. This form is considered more serious because it is often more difficult to deal with than stable angina. It may occur during exercise or emotional stress or in the absence of exertion. It can be very unpredictable, and it is not always relieved by rest as stable angina is. Sometimes unstable angina is a warning of an impending heart attack, although some people have unstable angina episodes for many years and never have a heart attack.

Another type of angina, which physicians usually call variant angina, often occurs during sleep. It is believed that this type is related to coronary spasm, another disorder, which is discussed later in this chapter.

When atherosclerosis reaches a point when a coronary artery, severely narrowed by a growing atheroma (plaque), is sealed off by a blood clot forming on the plaque or lodging in the narrowed area, a heart attack occurs. A blood clot is termed a *thrombus*; and the process is *coronary thrombosis*. Suddenly the part of the heart served by that artery is without its blood supply; in five minutes or less it may suffer severe damage or die.

A heart attack, medically termed a *myocardial infarction*, often produces symptoms that are similar to angina,

3. Heart Disease

but more intense. In a massive heart attack, the symptoms are frequently described as a very heavy, crushing feeling; the pain is centered under the breastbone. But some heart attack victims report pain in the back, between the shoulders, as well as in the left arm, jaw, shoulder, and back of the neck. Taking nitroglycerin or other angina medication usually does not relieve this pain. Sweating, shortness of breath, and nausea and vomiting also may be symptoms of a heart attack.

The so-called "silent" heart attacks, which the victim does not know he or she is having, are surprisingly common. Sometimes tests years later reveal that a patient has had one of these attacks. It may have been a mild attack with pain so slight that it was dismissed as indigestion or an aching muscle.

Mild heart attacks damage only a small area of the heart, and in many cases, when this damaged area heals, the heart is able to function as well as it did before the attack. But a major attack affects a larger area of the heart muscle, and it may hit a crucial area. For instance, if the attack interferes with the electrical pathways in the heart, it may cause abnormal heart rhythms, called *arrhythmias*, such as ventricular fibrillation. All the fibers in the ventricle contract independently, rather than together. The blood is not pumped out of the ventricle to where it is needed throughout the body. The heart ceases to do its job, and death is only moments away. If the victim is fortunate enough to have the heart attack in a hospital or an ambulance, a fibrillating heart often can be made to beat normally again with a powerful electrical stimulus from a defibrillator. But this machine is not readily available outside hospitals and ambulances, and defibrillation must be performed in a few minutes or the patient will die. A person trained in cardiopulmonary resuscitation (CPR) may be able to maintain a victim's circulation long enough for a defibrillator to be obtained.

A major heart attack may destroy such a large area of the heart that there is not enough healthy muscle left to do the heart's job properly. People in this condition are said to have heart failure.

Heart failure does not necessarily mean that the person afflicted with it is going to die soon. People with heart failure may live reasonably well for many years, but their hearts cannot pump enough blood to maintain the proper amount of blood in circulation, especially if exertion or emotional stress increase the body's demand for blood. Sometimes the cause is destroyed heart muscle; at other times it may be weak spots, or aneurysms, in the inner wall of the ventricles. When a heart attack damages enough tissue, the wall may become so weakened that it balloons out, creating a flexible sac like a blister. This loose sac, the aneurysm, absorbs much of the force of the heart's contractions. Every time the heart beats, some blood goes into the sac instead of moving out of the heart. The blood that ordinarily would be pumped out of the lungs and into the body backs up if the aneurysm is in the left ventricle. The lungs become partially filled with fluid, which may make breathing difficult and uncomfortable. If the damaged tissue is in

3. Heart Disease

the right ventricle, blood that would normally be drained out of the veins by the heart remains there and does not reach the lungs. The veins become congested and distended. The greater pressure pushes a watery fluid, blood without its red cells, into the tissues, usually the feet and ankles. The medical term for this condition is *edema*. The traditional popular term has been *dropsy*.

There are other causes of congestive heart failure besides a heart attack. Some of them are longstanding alcoholism or drug addiction; specific types of viral or bacterial infections, known as cardiomyopathies, that damage heart muscle; and hypertension. When the blood pressure in the vessels is too high, the heart is forced to pump against greater resistance. Eventually the heart muscle weakens. It becomes weaker with time and finally the heart gives out. Less commonly, this same process can be caused by fat-clogged arteries that produce a similar resistance.

If the heart failure is being caused by hypertension, a number of antihypertensive medications are commonly prescribed to help the patient. An individual may be advised to reduce physical activity to decrease the demands made on the heart, depending on his or her physical condition. Or the patient may be advised to increase physical activity so that exercise will strengthen the heart muscle and increase its pumping ability. A number of drugs, including digitalis, norepinephrine, dopamine, and glucanon, can be prescribed to reduce the frequency of the heartbeat and to strengthen each contraction of the heart.

Unlike heart attacks and hypertension, which mostly affect middle-aged and older adults, congestive heart failure also strikes infants, children, and younger adults. Some babies are born with defective hearts and circulatory vessels, congenital heart defects. The American Heart Association says that about eight out of every one thousand children born in this country have congenital heart disease. The causes of inborn heart defects are not known. Such drugs as LSD or thalidomide taken by a pregnant woman cause some defects in babies, and rare genetic disorders are also linked to some abnormalities. There is strong evidence that rubella, or German measles, is a major cause. If a mother contracts German measles in the first twelve weeks of pregnancy, the chances are better than one in twelve that she will give birth to a child with a defective heart. Most often, the aorta and the pulmonary artery are abnormally joined.

One of the most common congenital defects is a hole in the septum, the wall of muscle that separates the left and right sides of the heart. When the hole is between the two upper chambers (atria), it is called an atrial septal defect (ASD). When it is between the ventricles, it is a ventricular septal defect (VSD). In such cases, blood is moved between the two atria or the two ventricles. The pressure is greater on the heart's left side, so the blood is usually forced to the right side, where it is moved out to the lungs. However, if the pulmonary artery is blocked, the pressure is greater on the right side. Oxygen-deficient blood, in this case, is forced to the left side of the heart before it can pick up oxygen in the

3. Heart Disease

lungs. This oxygen-poor blood circulates through the aorta to the rest of the body. This blood is bluish, and it produces a bluish tinge in the skin and the lips. A common term for infants with this abnormality is *blue babies*.

Congestive heart failure in the young is also caused by rheumatic fever. The heart failure caused by this illness often occurs later, in the twenties, thirties, and forties. The damage caused by rheumatic fever may continue to scar certain heart valves over a period of years. Rheumatic heart disease is one of the most widespread cardiac disorders, affecting about 1.8 million Americans. Rheumatic fever is a reaction to a streptococcus infection; these bacteria can cause "strep throat." Streptococcus infection may affect the heart in any of three ways. The heart muscle may be injured; the lining of the heart (the endocardium) may be affected, particularly around the heart valves; and the sac in which the heart rests (the pericardium) may be damaged. Infection in any of these tissues makes the heart valves vulnerable to further infection years later if the person is exposed to certain microorganisms. The disease often scars and distorts the flaps of the valves. Sometimes the flaps thicken over time and lose their flexibility; then the valve obstructs the passage of blood or leaks, or both.

The valve most often damaged by rheumatic heart disease is the mitral valve, which regulates the flow of blood between the left atrium and the left ventricle. Usually the damaged valve sticks in a partly closed position, which diminishes the amount of blood that flows from the atrium down into the ventricle. In other cases, the valve sticks open and blood flows between the left atrium and the left ventricle. The first condition is called stenotic valve (*stenosis* is the medical term for tight or narrowed). Blood returning to the left atrium backs up, which causes the lungs to fill with fluid, a condition called pulmonary congestion. The patient has shortness of breath, which gets worse over time, until the patient has trouble breathing even when sitting or lying down.

If the aortic valve is stenotic, the left ventricle cannot pump enough blood into the aorta. There may not be enough blood passing through the aorta to the body's vital organs, including the heart and the brain. The patient experiences fatigue and lightheadedness, and eventually the heart may fail, making the condition worse.

A stenotic aorta may also be congenital (present at birth). The aortic valve may be narrowed; extra tissue may have built up just above the valve; or there may be a buildup of muscle tissue on the left ventricle just below this valve. Sometimes congenital aortic stenosis goes unnoticed for years until an obstructed valve produces symptoms of left ventricular failure.

Another common valve problem is insufficiency. Here the valve cusps may be too flexible or even floppy. Or conversely, they may be too stiff to close completely. When the mitral valve is "insufficient," some of the blood moving down into the left ventricle flows backward up into the left atrium. Then it must be pumped out again. If the aortic valve is insufficient, some of the blood in

3. Heart Disease

the aorta spills back into the ventricle. The term "heart murmur" describes the sound produced by this backward flow of blood through valves that do not close tightly. This backward blood flow is known as regurgitation.

Fortunately, most valve problems and congenital heart defects today can be successfully treated with medication or corrected by surgery. In many, many cases, people are helped to lead normal lives.

Still another heart problem is arrhythmia, or an abnormal heart rhythm. This problem was mentioned earlier in the chapter as a disorder that can result from a heart attack, but irregular heart rhythms can also be associated with heart valve and coronary artery disease. Irregular rhythms are also a common result of the normal aging process. As a person grows older, some of the electrical conduction fibers in the heart that help regulate the heartbeat may begin to wear out. This can cause a brief interruption in the signal relay.

The electrical current in the heart causes the chambers to contract and relax in rhythm, so when it is interrupted, the heart is no longer beating rhythmically. In cases when the heart beats too slowly, the condition is called bradycardia (a heart rate of less than sixty beats a minute). In cases where it beats too rapidly, the condition is called tachycardia (a heart rate of more than one hundred beats a minute). In some people, the heart rate becomes erratic (arrhythmic), swinging from bradycardia to tachycardia. The most dangerous arrhythmia is ventricular fibrillation, which was mentioned earlier in association with heart attacks. This erratic quivering of the heart muscle can lead to death if not treated immediately, usually by shocking the heart into a normal rhythm with a defibrillator.

Bradycardia is the most common disorder of the electrical conduction system. If the heart is beating more slowly than normal, not enough blood is transported to the body. The brain is affected first; dizziness, lightheadedness, fainting spells, blurred vision, and shortness of breath sometimes occur. With tachycardia, the most common symptom is a pounding sensation in the chest. The heart is not doing its job efficiently because it is contracting too rapidly to allow time for the ventricles to fill.

A separate cause of angina pains and heart attacks is coronary spasm. It often occurs in conjunction with the coronary artery disease known as atherosclerosis, though it is apparently unrelated. Even people with little or no atherosclerosis can have angina or heart attacks brought on by this strange phenomenon. When it happens, a segment of an artery, diseased or not, suddenly contracts long enough to obstruct blood flow to the heart muscle. The result is the same as that caused by atherosclerotic artery blockage. Yet when the spasm is over, there is no evidence that it has occurred. The chance of angina pain or a heart attack is, of course, increased if the artery in which the spasm occurs is already partially obstructed with plaque. A spasm can block it more readily than an undiseased artery. Medical science is still learning about the causes of coronary spasm. The evidence is not all in, but it is believed that emotional stress may be a cause. A coronary spasm can usually be relieved quickly by

3. Heart Disease

a nitroglycerin tablet, which opens up the blood vessels to increase the blood flow. Several newer medications, including Nifedipine and Verapamil, have proved to be very effective in preventing spasm.

We have discussed the many forms of heart disease and described the things that can go wrong with the heart and the blood circulation system. In Chapter Four, what medical science has learned about the origins of these ailments and the risks of contracting heart disease will be discussed.

4.
Look at Your Risk Factors

HEART DISEASE has been one of the most frustrating diseases for medical science to pin down with direct evidence of its causes. Even today, after many years of research, there is little scientific data to prove that eliminating the recognized risk factors of heart disease can reverse or prevent the disease. A vast body of medical observation, however, has been accumulating over the years, which points clearly and strongly to certain heart disease-associated factors. Hundreds of population studies have been conducted all over the world to see which traits, habits, and life-styles are common to victims of heart disease and to those who are not afflicted.

The largest, longest-running, and most important of these studies is the Framingham Heart Disease Epidemiology Study in the town of Framingham, Massachusetts. Framingham is typical of American communities of its size. Some of its 68,000 residents are executives

4. Look at Your Risk Factors 53

and white-collar workers in Boston, twenty miles away; other residents are factory workers and housewives.

In 1948, a group of physicians and scientists, including the famed cardiologist Dr. Paul Dudley White of the Harvard Medical School, launched an extraordinary investigation into the nature and causes of heart-related diseases. The effort, which became known as the Framingham Study, concentrated on stroke and heart failure, two of the most common circulatory ailments. The aim of the doctors was to compile a history of these illnesses by studying healthy people and seeing if there was a way to predict which ones would develop circulatory disorders.

The physicians began their quest for answers by following the health of every other local man and woman between the ages of thirty and sixty who had no symptoms of heart disease—a total of 5,127 residents. Later, the children of some of the original subjects were included in the study. The subjects were examined and measured for characteristics that might later be shown to relate to circulatory disease, and they were studied again every two years. This unique landmark in medical studies has gone on for nearly forty years.

After several decades of painstaking record-keeping and examination, the subjects of the Framingham Study were found to fall into two categories: those who had had heart attacks or strokes and those who had not yet been afflicted. The physicians studied the huge mass of statistics to find out what the victims had in common. A clear profile emerged. The people in the study who had suffered heart attacks or strokes smoked more cigarettes, lived with more emotional stress, weighed more, had higher blood pressure, were physically less active, and had greater amounts of cholesterol in their blood. The director of the study, Dr. William P. Castelli, concluded, "The average person headed for a premature heart attack or stroke is no mystery. These people can be identified."

These characteristics, which are probable causes of heart disease, are the habits, or the results of these habits, that people can control. Other probable causes (called risk factors) are beyond an individual's control. As a result of the Framingham Study, and a great many other studies with similar results, the majority of doctors today agree on a list of risk factors in heart disease. Perhaps the most important are smoking, hypertension, high blood lipids (cholesterol and other fats in the blood), and diabetes. Others are heredity (a history of heart disease in the family), obesity, a sedentary life-style, and emotional stress.

Some risk factors are beyond anyone's control: age (risk increases with age); sex (heart disease strikes men much more often than women); and a family history of heart disease. But the list of risk factors that *are* controllable is considerably longer: cigarette smoking; hypertension; high levels of cholesterol and other blood fats; diabetes; obesity; sedentary life-style; emotional stress; and sometimes personality type (the well-known type A), which contributes to emotional stress.

4. Look at Your Risk Factors

If each of these risk factors can lead to heart disease, then the risk is multiplied when the person has a combination of them, which many heart disease victims have. Some of them are interactive; for example, a sedentary life-style often leads to obesity, which, in turn, is sometimes associated with hypertension and high blood fats. The preponderance of evidence gained in the long-term Framingham Study, and in hundreds of other studies, strongly suggests that an individual can reduce his or her risk of heart disease by avoiding or controlling such risk factors as smoking, obesity, lack of exercise, emotional stress, hypertension, and high cholesterol and other blood fats. In people who already have heart disease, and perhaps have already had heart surgery, controlling or avoiding these risk factors can help them to reduce the symptoms of their disease and to live active lives with less pain and disability. It may help them to prolong a healthy life-style and avoid problems leading to repeat surgery for a longer time. Understanding these risk factors, and how they affect heart disease, may help you to control them yourself.

SMOKING

There is just about unanimous agreement among doctors that the most important controllable risk factor is cigarette smoking. Since this is a learned habit, it is possible to unlearn it. Possible but not necessarily easy! With all the publicity on the connection between smoking and lung cancer, many people would be surprised to learn that in the United States the risk of developing fatal heart disease is three times as great for cigarette smokers as the risk of cigarette smokers dying of lung cancer. Studies have shown repeatedly that if all other factors are equal, a smoker is twice as likely as a nonsmoker to have a heart attack and twice as likely to die from it. And it is also believed that smokers have a 50 percent greater risk of having a stroke than do nonsmokers. Heavier smokers are at greater risk. Some statistics show that men aged forty-five to fifty-four who smoke more than two packs of cigarettes a day have a ten times higher risk of dying of coronary heart disease than nonsmokers have. Most studies have indicated that pipe and cigar smokers have a lower risk than cigarette smokers, and one Canadian study indicated that the risk of heart disease for pipe and cigar smokers was no higher than for nonsmokers. But another study, in Switzerland, showed that pipe and cigar smokers, despite the fact that most of them do not inhale, do have a risk that is 50 percent greater than that of nonsmokers.

Women, who normally enjoy a lower risk of heart disease than men, lose that advantage when they smoke. And women who use oral contraceptives and also smoke increase their risk by as much as twenty times.

What makes smoking so dangerous? The ingredients of cigarette smoke are the culprits. About a dozen dangerous gases make up more than 90 percent of cigarette smoke. Carbon monoxide is the most important ingredient. The other 10 percent are particles, the most dangerous of which is nicotine. This is a poison. It has been

4. Look at Your Risk Factors

estimated that if the nicotine from five cigarettes was extracted and swallowed, it would cause death within a few minutes.

When nicotine is inhaled in cigarette smoke, it blocks some nerve impulses, the signals that stimulate muscles to relax and to contract. When it does this, it throws these impulses out of balance. This forces the smooth muscles of the small blood vessels to constrict, and this in turn, increases the blood pressure by increasing vascular resistance to the flow of blood. At the same time, nicotine increases the heart rate. Smoking just one or two cigarettes brings on this double effect, which lasts for fifteen to twenty minutes. Nicotine also interferes with the liver's ability to get rid of blood fats after a meal. This means that the fats that circulate in the bloodstream, instead of being disposed of by the liver, may contribute to the clogging of coronary arteries.

The other important ingredient of cigarette smoke—carbon monoxide—can make the effects of nicotine worse. Carbon monoxide interferes with the blood's oxygen delivery system. The hemoglobin molecule in red blood cells picks up oxygen in the lungs and transports it throughout the body. When carbon monoxide is inhaled, it enters the bloodstream and binds more strongly than oxygen with hemoglobin. This prevents the hemoglobin molecules from picking up oxygen. As a result, a heavy smoker may lose as much as 15 percent of the oxygen-carrying capacity of his or her red blood cells. Thus the heart and all the other parts of the body do not receive enough oxygen.

When the coronary arteries are already partially blocked by atherosclerosis, this can be dangerous. Since the rest of the body's tissues are not getting enough oxygen, the heart must pump faster to circulate blood through the lungs faster. The body tries to compensate for this oxygen deficiency by producing more red blood cells to increase the amount of hemoglobin, but these extra cells thicken the blood. And of course, thicker blood has a greater tendency to clot, which in itself is a danger in partially clogged arteries.

Another way in which carbon monoxide can cause damage is by altering the chemical activity of the cells that line the coronary arteries. Carbon monoxide makes the lining more porous, and this allows cholesterol to infiltrate the artery walls, which could trigger the buildup of fatty material in the artery.

Some smokers mistakenly believe that low-tar and low-nicotine cigarettes decrease the dangers of carbon monoxide. But carbon monoxide levels do not seem to correlate with tar and nicotine levels. Standards of maximum safe levels of carbon monoxide have been established for the air in factories to protect workers' health. If you are a heavy smoker, even of low-tar and low-nicotine cigarettes, you are inhaling carbon monoxide at levels eight times higher than the maximum allowable level in factories.

Clearly this primary risk of smoking is dangerous to your heart's health. If you have been a smoker for years, you may feel it is too late to stop now that the damage has already been done. But medical science has evidence

4. Look at Your Risk Factors

to show that your chances of avoiding heart disease can improve dramatically if you stop smoking. The risk to your heart and arteries can be reversed over a period of time, and the time is probably shorter than you think. For example, it only takes about two weeks for the red blood cells to become free of carbon monoxide. Framingham Study statistics indicate that former smokers can cut their risks of heart disease in half within two years. And within ten or fifteen years, these ex-smokers' chances of dying of a heart attack are about the same as those of nonsmokers, that is, people who have never smoked. If you already have heart disease, you may believe you have already lost the ballgame, but doctors know in your case it is all the more important to stop smoking. By doing so, you can lessen the risk of further damage to your arteries and heart and increase your chances of living with fewer heart disease symptoms. You can't lose.

HYPERTENSION

The most prevalent heart and blood vessel disease is hypertension (high blood pressure), which affects an estimated 8 to 18 percent of adults in the industrialized countries of the world. It may very well be the most dangerous, too, because it usually strikes without symptoms, and, in combination with other heart and blood vessel diseases, it threatens life and health. Hypertension is often associated with stroke. Under great pressure, the blood pounds against the brain's blood vessel walls until it roughens them and wears the vessels out. Ironically, this most common affliction is not well understood by the general public. Many people mistakenly take the term *hypertension* to mean *nervous tension*, and they are surprised to learn that calm people can have hypertension, too.

The force with which the blood pushes against the walls of blood vessels varies during each heartbeat. When the heart contracts to pump blood, the blood pressure rises to its highest level (the systolic pressure). Then when the heart relaxes, the blood pressure drops to its lowest level (the diastolic pressure).

What determines blood pressure levels is a complicated combination of bodily actions. If you look at these factors in groups, the first group consists of physical factors: the volume of blood in the body, the volume that can be pumped by the heart with each beat, and the resistance the blood meets as it is expelled through the aorta and moves through smaller and smaller blood vessels.

Another group consists of chemical actions in the body. Substances produced by some glands and organs are released in the bloodstream, to affect the circulatory system. The adrenal glands, which sit on top of the kidneys, release epinephrine (adrenaline) and norepinephrine (noradrenaline). These hormones stimulate the heart so that it pumps harder, and they also cause some blood vessels to constrict. There is another adrenal hormone, aldosterone, that causes the body to retain salt and water. This has the effect of increasing the volume of blood, which also affects the blood pressure. The kidneys

4. Look at Your Risk Factors

also produce an enzyme, renin, that reacts with certain substances in the bloodstream to form angiotensin I and angiotensin II, which also cause cardiovascular changes.

Blood pressure is also regulated to some extent by another group of factors, the workings of the autonomic nervous system. This system controls the functions we don't consciously control, like heartbeat, breathing, and digestion. A group of nerve cells, the baroreceptors, monitor the blood pressure the way thermostats monitor heat in a house. These cells are the body's means of regulating these functions. If the blood pressure varies considerably, the baroreceptors sense the change and emit electrical impulses that "tell" the heart and blood vessels to return to a normal state.

Any of these regulators may malfunction, and when this happens, the blood pressure changes, usually by increasing. Among the physical governing factors that may change are the arteries, which, already narrowed by fat deposits, become even narrower. This increases the resistance to blood flow, much in the way that a nozzle at the end of a water hose restricts the flow of water through the hose. When this happens, the water pressure within the hose—and, similarly, the blood pressure within an artery—increases. The chemical regulators of blood pressure might be affected by tumors of the adrenal glands so that the adrenal produces greater than usual amounts of epinephrine, norepinephrine, or aldosterone and this increases the blood pressure. Diseased kidneys may secrete increased amounts of renin, which can also increase blood pressure.

In other cases, the nerve regulators, or baroreceptors, may fail to do their job, in effect telling the body that blood pressure is normal when it is really too high. This type of disorder is relatively rare. Doctors can usually identify these causes of high blood pressure, but in most cases it is impossible to tell which of the regulators is malfunctioning or why. These cases of hypertension are called "essential" hypertension, a medical term that means the cause cannot be determined.

Blood pressure is measured with a device bearing the tongue-tripping name *sphygmomanometer*, the standard inflatable cuff seen in medical offices and hospitals everywhere. The device measures pressure inside the major artery in the arm when the cuff is inflated and thus tightened. The numbers in a blood pressure reading represent the height, in millimeters, of a column of mercury that the air in the cuff can raise in a tube. In a blood pressure of 120/80, the systolic pressure in the arteries is sufficient to support a column of mercury 120 millimeters high, and diastolic pressure, 80 millimeters.

One blood pressure reading may not reveal the true blood pressure, because pressure changes in response to a number of factors. For example, if you were late for your medical appointment and hurried to the doctor's office, the exertion might raise your blood pressure temporarily. Similarly, anxiety over the medical examination can also raise blood pressure. Most doctors prefer to take at least two readings at intervals to get a more accurate picture of your blood pressure.

4. Look at Your Risk Factors

But not all doctors, hospitals, and research studies view blood pressure levels in exactly the same way. Thus one physician may consider a reading normal and another may view it as elevated. There is a consensus among medical experts that recognizes blood pressure of 120/80 as normal and desirable for a healthy adult man or woman. A level of 140/90 is generally regarded as the point at which hypertension occurs and at which many physicians decide that a patient needs medical care to control it. At higher levels, especially those over 160/95, there is the almost universal medical opinion that that level of hypertension is dangerous. There are borderline values between the normal figures and the high figures.

Medical experts generally agree that when blood pressure is higher than the normal level of 120/80, the heart must pump harder than it normally would to circulate the blood through the body. This condition may produce heart failure over a period of time. Also, hypertension seems to encourage fatty deposits to build up faster than they normally would in the coronary arteries. This, of course, may block the arteries totally at some point, depriving the heart of its vital supply of blood. And hypertension can injure and weaken blood vessels in the brain, which leads to strokes, as well as in the kidneys and eyes, which lead to kidney failure and blindness, respectively.

The effects of hypertension may differ in individual patients, but overall, there is plenty of medical evidence to show the damage it does. The statistics compiled over many years in the Framingham Study indicate that risks of death or disability from stroke, coronary artery disease, or kidney failure increased considerably as soon as the blood pressure of the people in the study rose above 120/80. And the actuarial studies of insurance companies have shown the same thing: as blood pressure rises, so do risks of heart disease and stroke. At the same time, life expectancy is lowered.

Fortunately doctors today are able to lower blood pressure to less threatening levels in about 85 percent of hypertensive patients. There are a number of ways to do this, but the patient must cooperate. Overweight people can lose weight, which makes the heart's pumping job easier. Smokers can quit smoking, thereby eliminating the nicotine in tobacco smoke that constricts blood vessels and raises blood pressure.

Hypertensive patients may also be advised to reduce their salt intake. The sodium in salt causes the body to retain fluids, which increases the total volume of blood in circulation and thus raises the blood pressure. A drastically reduced salt intake helps to lower blood pressure in some cases.

Exercise programs (which should be medically supervised) can also help to lower blood pressure. So can relaxation periods during the working day and at night, as well as on days off.

For people who cannot lower their blood pressure enough through these means, many effective drugs have

4. Look at Your Risk Factors

been developed in recent years. Your doctor may prescribe one drug or a combination of drugs to treat you. Some antihypertensive medicines cause side effects in some people, including weakness, sleepiness, digestive upsets, and sexual problems, but not all patients have such side effects, and your doctor will try to find the medication that works best for you. One of the most common, helpful drugs is the diuretic. Diuretics cause the body to excrete more water and sodium than usual, which reduces the total blood volume and pressure. Sometimes diuretics are used in combination with other medication.

Vasodilators, such as hydralazine and diazoxide, are often prescribed along with diuretics. These drugs affect the walls of the blood vessels directly, causing them to relax and enlarge. This, of course, lowers the resistance to the blood flow and lowers the blood pressure.

Another group of drugs, the sympatholytics, interfere with the chemical nerve signals that help to control blood pressure. Reserpine, a tranquilizer, interferes with nerve impulses to the adrenal glands so these glands produce fewer of the hormones that increase blood pressure. There are also newer sympatholytics, such as guanethidine, clonidine, and a group known as beta blockers. The drugs in the last group, which include propranolol and metoprolol, affect the nerve endings called beta receptors. Some beta receptors help control the release of the pressure-regulating hormones; others affect the strength and speed of the heartbeat.

Beta blockers dull these receptors, causing blood pressure to drop.

If you have hypertension, you will probably need to take your antihypertensive medicine for the rest of your life. Some people are tempted to stop taking the medication when they feel better, but to do so is to remove your protection against coronary heart disease, stroke, and congestive heart failure, diseases hypertension can cause.

Until recently, many physicians were somewhat reluctant to prescribe medications for mild or borderline cases of hypertension. With the possible side effects and the expense, they were not sure the benefits were worth the cost of the treatment. But a five-year study, completed in 1979 by the National Heart, Lung and Blood Institute, provided solid scientific evidence that drug treatment could save lives even for people with mild hypertension.

In the study, the Hypertension Detection and Follow-Up Program, nearly 159,000 Americans between the ages of thirty and sixty-nine were screened. The researchers chose about 11,000 subjects with diastolic pressure (the lower of the recorded pressures) above 90 and divided them into three groups: those with diastolic pressures between 90 and 104, those with pressures between 105 and 114, and those with pressures above 115. Approximately one-half of the patients in each category were sent to their physicians or local clinics for traditional care. The other one-half in each group were treated with a variety of drugs designed to reduce diastolic pressure to a point somewhere below 90. Com-

4. Look at Your Risk Factors

binations of drugs were tried, and some patients received up to four medications simultaneously.

The results in each of the designated groups were convincing. Among the patients in the drug-treated half, there were 17 percent fewer deaths after five years than there were in the half referred to private doctors and clinics. There were almost 45 percent fewer deaths from stroke and about 26 percent fewer deaths from heart attacks. An even more surprising result was that drugs lowered the death rate among patients with what is often considered mild hypertension—those with diastolic pressures of 90 to 105—by some 20 percent overall. Stroke fatalities dropped 45 percent and heart attack deaths dropped 46 percent. Dr. Jeremiah Stamler, a member of the study's data evaluation committees, stated, "For the first time, we have clear evidence of the efficacy of therapy in so-called mild hypertension."

Though the study results were encouraging for the treatment of a great many cases, the conclusion does not mean that drug therapy is automatically the treatment of choice in all cases of hypertension. The side effects of medication vary widely in individual patients, and physicians have found that in many cases, nondrug therapy, which emphasizes weight reduction, exercises, relaxation, and restriction of sodium, is more desirable than drug therapy.

Meanwhile, research on hypertension continues. At the Cleveland Clinic Foundation, which has been a leader in hypertension and cardiovascular research, the effort commands a high priority. More than forty years ago,

Irvine H. Page, M.D., emeritus director of the Division of Research, laid the intellectual foundation for the knowledge that exists today of the "regulators" described earlier in this chapter that affect blood pressure. Dr. Page viewed the factors associated with hypertension as a "mosaic," with interrelated pieces. His mosaic theory, which is still applicable and useful today, lists the most important factors researchers consider in association with high blood pressure: genetic, environmental, anatomical, adaptive, neural, endocrine, humoral, and hemodynamic.

Knowing that there was no single cause of most hypertension, Dr. Page realized that unraveling such a complex, multifaceted problem required a multidisciplinary approach by scientists and clinicians. He gathered such a group of experts at the Cleveland Clinic, and the result has been a series of important discoveries in hypertension research over many years. Researchers here, including F. Merlin Bumpus, Ph.D., an organic chemist, and James W. McCubbin, M.D., were the first to purify and synthesize the hormone angiotensin and to identify some of its complex actions.

Discovered in the late thirties by Dr. Page and his colleagues in Cleveland and by Eduardo Braun-Menendez and his colleagues in Argentina, angiotensin has a significant role in a very important regulatory pathway: The human kidney responds to a drop in blood pressure by secreting renin, which activates the angiotensin present in the bloodstream. The angiotensin raises blood

4. Look at Your Risk Factors

pressure by multiple means. It contracts the muscles in the arterial walls, increases the heart rate and the force of the cardiac contractions, and stimulates the adrenal glands to release aldosterone. The hormone aldosterone causes the body to retain salt and water, which increases the blood volume and thus the blood pressure.

With the synthesis of angiotensin by Dr. Bumpus and co-investigators in 1956, the search for chemicals to block the hormone began. Researchers at the Cleveland Clinic were the first to develop a successful blocker.

The discovery was most welcome, as the problem of finding drugs that control blood pressure with few side effects has haunted doctors and researchers since Dr. Page's early research. Today, side effects continue to be the main reason patients resist therapy.

"That most hypertensives feel no symptoms compounds the problem," says Donald G. Vidt, M.D., head of Clinical Hypertension in the Department of Hypertension and Nephrology at the Cleveland Clinic Foundation. "When a patient is screened and first learns he has high blood pressure, he may be feeling perfectly well. So he's surprised to learn he has a disease that can shorten his life. Then he has to take a medication which may make him feel less well because of its side effects. On top of that, he may have to take medication for the rest of his life—in 98 percent of the cases, hypertension can only be controlled, not cured.

"With hypertension it is important that patients become partners in their care. They have to be educated about their disease and informed of their risks if the blood pressure is not controlled adequately. We feel strongly that patients should know about the drugs they take and how each acts. We also encourage home blood pressure measurement."

"About a quarter of the hypertensives in America remain unidentified," says Ray W. Gifford, Jr., M.D., chairman of the Cleveland Clinic's Department of Hypertension and Nephrology, "even after more than a decade of national health campaigns. Another 40 percent does not control the hypertension adequately." Controlling even mild hypertension is important because over one-half the deaths attributable to hypertension occurs in the 70 percent of patients who are mildly hypertensive.

Dr. Gifford has been part of a National High Blood Pressure Coordinating Committee subgroup that aims at redefining risk levels. Based on the study of the best epidemiological data available, the group recommends that three levels of risk be established. The emphasis is on informing those people with intermediate levels of risk of the life-style changes they might adopt to prevent further increases in blood pressure.

"We did not want to create arbitrary labels that might cause panic or can be used to stigmatize, say, someone applying for a job," says Dr. Gifford. "At the same time, the group with diastolic readings between 80 and 89 might consider weight control, giving up smoking, using less salt and making other dietary changes to reduce risks. Also, they should monitor their blood pres-

4. Look at Your Risk Factors

sure more closely in the future because elevated blood pressure engenders even higher blood pressures with time."

The group recommends adoption of these risk levels:

Minimal risk is associated with diastolic blood pressures under 80 millimeters of mercury (80 mm Hg). Blood pressure contributes little if at all to these people's risk of disease and death.

Intermediate risk is associated with diastolic pressures of 80 to 89 mm Hg. These people experience a risk twice that of the minimal risk group.

Higher risk is experienced by those with diastolic pressures of 90 mm Hg or higher and/or systolic pressures of 160 mm Hg or higher. These people should be reevaluated for possible treatment.

Based on these risk categories, 41 percent of the adult U.S. population would belong to the minimal risk category, 34 percent to the intermediate risk category, and 25 percent to the higher risk category. Though effective treatment is available to minimize the complications of hypertension, high blood pressure has yet to gain the popular recognition it should have. It remains the most prevalent risk factor contributing to premature heart disease in this country.

CHOLESTEROL

The role of cholesterol in coronary heart disease has been debated by medical scientists for decades. There is a great deal of evidence linking the two, but it could be considered "circumstantial" because there is no laboratory proof of the process whereby consumption of dietary cholesterol is a direct cause of heart disease. However, the evidence is persuasive enough to convince many scientists that the fat levels in the diets of people in industrial countries should be lowered to reduce heart disease.

Cholesterol, a waxy, yellowish material, is an essential ingredient of all the body's organs because it is a structural part of all cell walls. It aids in the formation of bile acids for digestion and in the production of hormones. But in contrast to these "good" functions, it also is implicated in gallstone formation and anemia, as well as atherosclerosis. Cholesterol is carried in the bloodstream, and this is where it is believed to cause trouble for the coronary arteries. Many studies have indicated that the higher the cholesterol level in the blood, the greater the risk of coronary heart disease.

But in recent years, medical scientists have discovered that total blood cholesterol level is not a reliable measure of risk. They have found that cholesterol has different components, and at least one of these components seems to protect against heart disease. There is a greater knowledge today of all types of blood fats, including the triglycerides, which make up 98 to 99 percent of the weight of food fats. Neither cholesterol nor the triglycerides dissolve in water. This means that in an unaltered state they cannot be transported in the bloodstream, which is principally water. But in the body, these blood fats are

4. Look at Your Risk Factors

joined with proteins to form molecules that are soluble in water. These special molecules, which transport fats in the blood, are the lipoproteins.

Lipoproteins are classified, according to their density, into four main groups. Those with the lowest density pick up triglycerides from food fats. They are then up to 95 percent triglyceride, with only a small amount of cholesterol.

The next lightest group, the very low density lipoproteins (VLDLs), carry only about 15 percent of the cholesterol present in the blood.

The next heaviest group, the low density lipoproteins (LDLs), are suspected of being troublemakers. They carry about 65 percent of the cholesterol present in the blood.

The last group, the high density lipoproteins (HDLs), transport only about 20 percent of the cholesterol in the blood. Researchers believe that HDLs are the "good" cholesterol fraction because they pick up other cholesterol from the bloodstream and carry it to the liver for breakdown and subsequent removal from the body. Another theory suggests that HDLs interfere with the absorption of the "bad" LDL cholesterol within artery wall cells.

No matter what the explanation, there is abundant evidence from numerous studies that HDL levels do have an effect on risk of heart disease. In the past decade, statistics from several studies saw low HDL levels as a warning sign of increased risk of heart disease. And conversely, the higher the HDL level, the lower the risk. In the Framingham Study, the average man had an HDL level of 45 (measured in milligrams per 100 milliliters), whereas the average woman had a level of 55. The difference may help to explain why women have a lower heart attack rate. Researchers have calculated that for every five points the HDL level is below the average level of 45, there is a 25 percent increase in the risk of heart disease.

But if HDL levels play an important role in the risk of heart disease, then conversely, LDL levels are also important. These cholesterol-laden lipoproteins are believed to carry much of the fatty substances that lodges in coronary arteries to block blood flow. So high levels of LDL indicate a higher risk of heart disease. And the level of total cholesterol in the blood is still important because people with high total cholesterol levels usually have high LDL levels as well.

Evidence linking high total cholesterol levels with increased risk of heart disease has been accumulating for years. Some scientists and physicians still disagree with the notion that lowering total cholesterol levels can reduce the incidence of heart disease, but the vast majority of medical experts believe that cholesterol level is important.

The general consensus among physicians and scientists is this: It is known that most heart attack and stroke victims have arteries clogged with cholesterol and that the amount of blood cholesterol to create such blockages

4. Look at Your Risk Factors

can be affected by the fats in the food eaten. This is not, in itself, solid proof that a high blood cholesterol level causes heart disease or stroke, nor is it proof that consumption of fat is crucial in determining the blood cholesterol level. There could be other influences, and scientists are still trying to learn more about them. For example, culture, which affects the types of activities people engage in, could have an adverse or a favorable effect on some individuals. Genetic characteristics, which differ considerably among the many ethnic and racial groups of the world, could also play a part in determining heart disease risk.

Studies are being undertaken all over the world as medical scientists continue to search for the answers to these questions. Some of the studies observe and compare groups of people with different diets; other studies observe one group of people whose diet is changing. In other research, experiments with animals explore the process by which diet may produce atherosclerosis.

One of the best-known, widest-ranging studies comparing national differences in diet and their correlation with heart disease took place about three decades ago. It was the Seven Countries Coronary Disease Study, organized by Dr. Ancel Keys of the University of Minnesota. The seven countries were the United States, Finland, the Netherlands, Italy, Yugoslavia, Greece, and Japan. The study's results helped focus attention on the role of diet and cholesterol in heart disease; a clear connection was shown in each country between heart attacks and average cholesterol level in the blood. And equally important, the cholesterol level in the blood and the amount of saturated fat in a country's typical diet could be connected.

The Seven Countries Study showed that the Japanese, who had the lowest heart attack rate of the countries studied, consumed the smallest amount of saturated fat —only about 3 percent of all the calories in their typical diet. The people of Finland, the country with the highest heart attack rate, consumed the greatest amount of saturated fats. Their high consumption of butter, cheese, milk, and sausage brought their total saturated fats to about 20 percent of their total calories. These results certainly suggest that diet plays a key role in cholesterol levels and occurrence of heart disease, but they do not rule out racial differences or cultural influences.

Do the inherited characteristics of race matter? Science is still trying to find out. There is evidence from a number of studies that suggests that racial differences may not matter. These studies have followed people who have migrated from their native, low-heart-disease-risk countries to high-risk countries. People who move to another country usually start eating the foods common in that culture. If racial origin were the key risk factor, a change in diet should have no effect on these peoples' coronary risks. But a change in diet *does* change the coronary risks, as is shown in a number of studies. For example, one study followed Japanese who moved to California and showed that they had ten times as much coronary heart disease as Japanese who still lived in

4. Look at Your Risk Factors

Japan. Other studies concentrated on Italians who moved to New York, Irish who moved to Boston, and Jews from Yemen who migrated to Israel. In each instance, the move was from relatively low-risk countries to high-risk ones. And in every study, the incidence of heart disease increased significantly after the subjects migrated and changed their diets.

Other studies of native inhabitants of high-risk countries who do not adhere to the typical diets of those countries have shown similar results. In the United States, studies have shown that Seventh Day Adventists, who eat a vegetarian diet, have less than one-half the heart attack rate of American men on the average. Another study, led by Dr. Edward Kass of Harvard Medical School, examined eighteen small communes of vegetarians living in Boston. The men in these groups had incredibly low blood pressures, an average of 110/62, compared with the U.S. average of 131/83. The cholesterol levels of the subjects were equally impressive—an average of 125, about one-half the American average. Considering that the long-term Framingham Study showed that people with cholesterol levels of about 260 have four times the incidence of cardiovascular disease as people with levels at or below 220, the potential risk-lowering of a vegetarian diet is impressive indeed.

Medical scientists have been looking for the hopeful evidence of people lowering both their cholesterol levels and their incidence of heart disease, and there are some study results. A twelve-year study in Finland showed that men who reduced the cholesterol in their diet for six years cut their rate of death from heart attacks in half. When the subjects went back to their former diet, the coronary death rate climbed again. A similar study in Norway found that more than 1,200 men with abnormally high cholesterol levels cut their heart attack rate nearly in half when they switched to a low-cholesterol diet. The evidence goes on and on, study after study.

Yet in the face of this "circumstantial" but persuasive evidence, there is still some controversy about the role of diet and cholesterol. Because science is still learning about the role of heredity and other factors in heart disease, some research experts are not convinced that diet has as much influence on the disease as others believe it has. A few years ago, the Food and Nutrition Board of the National Academy of Sciences concluded that diet and cholesterol were not the key factors and that there were other factors operating within the body, which are still not sufficiently understood, that very likely were more decisive in determining whether heart disease will occur. But an impressive number of experts disagreed—scientists at the American Heart Association, the Harvard School of Public Health, and the U.S. Department of Health, Human Services, and of Agriculture, to name some—and vehemently argued their views that the evidence for the role of cholesterol in heart disease is overwhelming. This is the majority view in medicine today. To be fair, the opponents of the cholesterol theory do have some evidence they can point to in support of their beliefs. Not all study results have fitted neatly into

4. Look at Your Risk Factors

a pattern that would indicate cholesterol's role in heart disease. One of the puzzling things about the medical research is the fact that some results (in a minority of studies) contradict the majority of study results. For example, in some clinical trials carried out in New York, Los Angeles, London, Oslo, and Helsinki, selected groups of people were kept on diets low in saturated fat. Their cholesterol levels and rates of death were compared with those of other groups of people whose diets differed only in fat content. The results showed that the people on the low-fat diets did, indeed, have lower cholesterol levels than the groups with more fat intake, but the difference in death rates between the paired groups was insignificant—a disappointing finding.

Probably the most important evidence in support of the view that cholesterol levels have an effect on heart disease and death from such disease came in 1984. This was the culmination of a ten-year, $150 million study conducted by the National Heart, Lung and Blood Institute. This major study followed 3,806 men, ages thirty-five to fifty-nine, who had cholesterol levels in their blood of at least 265 milligrams, well above the national average of 215 milligrams. One-half of these men were given six daily doses of cholestyramine, a drug that lowers cholesterol in the blood. The other one-half were given similar doses of a placebo, which did not contain the drug.

The results were encouraging. They indicated that the men who took the cholesterol-lowering cholestyramine over the ten-year period had a drop in serum cholesterol of 8.5 percent, suffered 19 percent fewer heart attacks, experienced 21 percent fewer coronary bypass operations, and most important, had a 24 percent lower death rate than the men who did not receive the cholesterol-lowering drug. The conclusion was that for every 1 percent drop in blood cholesterol, there is a 2 percent reduction in heart disease. Another result worth noting was that the drug-treated group averaged 12.6 percent lower low density cholesterol (LDL), which is considered the most harmful component of cholesterol.

"This is the first study to demonstrate conclusively that the risk of coronary heart disease can be reduced by lowering blood cholesterol, as we previously suspected," said Basil M. Rifkind, M.D., of the National Heart, Lung and Blood Institute.

Robert L. Levy, M.D., of Columbia University, who headed the National Heart, Lung and Blood Institute when the study began, said the results have implications far beyond the middle-aged men with high cholesterol levels used in the study.

"Now, for the first time, we have conclusive evidence that people can do something about heart disease by lowering their cholesterol," Dr. Levy stated. Some experts estimate that more than 40 million Americans have moderate-to-high blood cholesterol levels. If all of them reduced these levels to normal, some experts believe, perhaps 100,000 deaths could be prevented each year. That is why most doctors advise patients with significant

4. Look at Your Risk Factors

coronary risk factors to modify their eating habits to reduce the amount of cholesterol and saturated fats they consume. Until final proof is established, it seems to be a prudent course.

DIABETES

When the disease diabetes mellitus occurs, the body fails to produce the amount of insulin it needs. The pancreas manufactures insulin, a hormone used by the body to metabolize sugar and other carbohydrates. If an insufficient amount of insulin is produced, sugar accumulates in the blood. One of the problems of higher blood sugar levels is that such levels raise the level of cholesterol in the blood, which can lead to early atherosclerosis.

Medical science has not yet determined the cause of diabetes, but it is believed to be inherited, at least in some people. It has been shown that people who develop diabetes early in life have a greater risk of developing coronary heart disease than people who develop diabetes in their later years. It has been found that overweight people are more likely to develop diabetes than thinner people, because their cells do not respond as well to the insulin produced by the pancreas. It is possible to keep diabetes under control with proper medicine, diet, and weight control. Medical experts are not yet sure whether this will help prevent atherosclerosis, but there is some evidence that suggests that it does.

OBESITY

The word *obese* has an ugly connotation, conjuring up images of people who are vastly overweight. But to doctors, obesity is a term that can be applied to a great many people who do not think of themselves as "fat." Medical experts know that even mild obesity is a risk factor in heart disease and in other ailments.

A fourteen-member panel of health officials from a variety of disciplines was convened by the National Institutes of Health to try to arrive at a consensus on current knowledge about the dangers to health of various levels of obesity. The panel announced its conclusions in 1985. Any level of obesity increases health risks, the panel noted, but it singled out a level of 20 percent or more above "desirable" body weight as the point at which otherwise healthy adults should be treated.

In defining obesity, the panel used the 1983 Metropolitan Life Insurance Company Table (which is itself controversial because the levels for desirable weight in it are higher than the company's 1959 table), based on the weights at which death rates are the lowest among people with life insurance policies.

According to this table, an adult man who is 5 feet 10 inches tall and 20 percent overweight would weigh 192 pounds, and an adult woman who is 5 feet 4 inches tall and 20 percent overweight would weight 160 pounds.

However, according to data compiled in the long-running Framingham Study, a lesser degree of obesity, even 10 percent or less, can impair health. Dr. Castelli,

4. Look at Your Risk Factors

the director of the Framingham Study, has concluded, "Obesity is as powerful a risk factor as any that we know, including smoking and high blood pressure." Many physicians define obesity as being 10 percent heavier than the ideal weight for a particular height and frame. Extra weight increases the strain on the heart. If a person is extremely obese, the heart muscle may contain so much fat that its ability to contract is impaired. Medical studies have shown that obesity can be an important predictor of heart disease, particularly in younger people.

Aside from its own harmful effects on the heart, obesity is an important risk because it increases the effects of other risk factors. Overweight people are more likely to have hypertension, high blood cholesterol levels, and diabetes. Overweight people are also more likely to have low levels of high density lipoproteins (HDL), the "good" cholesterol believed to protect against atherosclerosis. And finally, because overweight people often find it harder to move around easily, they avoid exercise and become increasingly sedentary—a life-style that is also a risk factor in coronary heart disease.

THE SEDENTARY LIFE-STYLE

Before automobile transportation became commonplace, our great-grandparents got more daily exercise than most of us get today. They had to walk much more. They also exercised more because more physical labor was involved in housework (without today's appliances) and in many jobs. There is no way to calculate the other risk factors involved, of course, but the fact is that heart disease was nowhere near as prevalent then as it is now. How much did exercise protect our ancestors against heart disease? That cannot be quantified, either, but it is known that exercise and activity are important in maintaining a healthy heart and good blood circulation. And more than one-half the adults in the United States follow a sedentary life-style and take very little exercise. A sedentary life-style and obesity seem to go together—another example of risk factors interacting.

Frequent exercise strengthens the heart muscle because the heart must pump more blood. The stronger the heart muscle, the more blood it pumps per beat, so it is not required to beat as often. Exercise also helps reduce stress because it lowers the level of those hormones that increase the heart rate and elevate blood pressure. What is more, exercise has been shown to increase the level of high density lipoproteins (HDL) in the blood, a beneficial factor in reducing the risk of heart disease. And of course, it can help people lose weight, which helps lower the previously mentioned risk factors of hypertension, high blood cholesterol levels, and diabetes. With a sedentary life-style, some of these potential benefits are lost.

How *much* you lose cannot be determined because lack of exercise is only one risk factor and must be considered in combination with other factors. In some studies, a reduction in coronary heart disease in people who exercise regularly has been demonstrated. Perhaps the

4. Look at Your Risk Factors

best-known of these is an eighteen-year study of nearly 17,000 male alumni of Harvard University. Headed by Dr. Ralph Paffenbarger, a Stanford University epidemiologist, the study included men who entered Harvard between 1916 and 1950. A report based on the study findings was published in the *Journal of the American Medical Association* in 1984.

The study showed that exercise was associated with fewer deaths from a wide range of causes, most notably cardiac and respiratory diseases. The strongest relationship was established for cardiovascular disease, which was reduced substantially for study group members who expended at least 2,000 calories weekly in walking, climbing, and athletics. The researchers found that the statistically adjusted death rates of the least active men were nearly twice as high as they were for those subjects who expended the minimum of 2,000 calories a week. One of the study's findings was that a member of the study group who converted from a sedentary to an active life-style could reduce his coronary heart disease by 33 percent. How much exercise is involved in expending 2,000 calories a week? Brisk walking typically burns about 400 calories an hour, whereas jogging expends approximately 500 to 600 calories an hour.

"If everyone in the study had been physically active, there would have been a 23 percent lower incidence of coronary disease," Dr. Paffenbarger concluded. "People who are physically active live longer."

But the role of exercise in preventing coronary heart

disease is still controversial; many physicians do not accept the study's findings as definitive. Epidemiological studies remain "suggestive" rather than conclusive, many experts say, because of the selection factor: people who are already healthy might be more likely to exercise.

Physicians who treat cardiac patients every day see plenty of exceptions to the general findings of studies. Dr. Shirey, a veteran cardiologist on the staff of the Cleveland Clinic, puts the role of exercise in perspective. "I recommend appropriate exercise to cardiac patients because it generally does offer a number of benefits," he says. "Sometimes the symptoms of coronary heart disease, such as chest pain, can be reduced when a patient becomes more active. Exercise may foster the growth of collateral vessels and improve function of the heart muscle. It is also helpful in lowering other risk factors such as hypertension and obesity. But exercise alone is not the answer to reducing coronary risk. It must be considered only one of several risk factors, and not the most important one at that. I know some people who are eighty-five years old and they have been sedentary for their entire adult lives. They happen to have the right heredity and other factors which have protected them from heart disease."

Although Dr. Shirey and most other physicians recommend exercise, they caution that it should be moderate exercise, geared to the individual's condition. Many physicians believe that daily walking is one of the most effective forms of exercise and that it is preferable to

4. Look at Your Risk Factors

overly strenuous activities such as running and certain competitive sports. So moderation may be the key to being active and avoiding a sedentary life-style.

EMOTIONAL STRESS

Emotional stress, or more accurately, the individual's *reaction* to emotional stress, is another risk factor that is hard to measure and quantify. However, practicing physicians know from experience with many patients that it is a real risk factor in coronary heart disease. Whereas some people seem to thrive on high-pressure, fast-paced life-styles, others suffer physical consequences because of how they react to stressful situations. It is difficult to measure stress, because the feelings people associate with stress range from slight annoyance and frustration to intense anger, but it is known that stress produces physical changes in the human body.

In stressful situations, the body is alerted by the brain to react involuntarily. Epinephrine is quickly produced by the adrenal, an endocrine gland. The hormone is the body's way of preparing itself for "fight or flight," as this involuntary reaction is commonly called. Some muscles immediately become tense, the heart beats faster so it can pump more blood to the muscles, and the blood pressure rises. These physical responses play an important role in helping the body prepare for stressful situations, particularly those requiring physical action. The problem is, many of the stressful situations we face today do not require a physical response. And if they are chronic situations, such as unhappiness on the job, an unhappy marriage or other emotional relationship, or, say, a long-term family illness, the stress reaction can damage the heart and the blood vessels.

Physicians who have treated thousands of cardiac patients recognize stress as an important factor in coronary heart disease. Dr. Shirey says, "It's difficult to measure the effect, but I don't think we get away with too much stress. We pay for it. Stress can elevate the blood pressure to harmful levels, and it may cause chemical actions that can be injurious to our arteries. It may play a role in coronary spasms. I think we need to avoid and reduce stress in our lives as much as we can."

PERSONALITY TYPE

There is a theory, believed by many physicians, that certain personality types may be especially prone to developing heart disease. "There are the overly ambitious, high-powered executive types with heart disease," says Dr. Shirey. "These patients are very competitive, have a sense of time urgency, are perfectionists, and generally are people who are determined to do too many things in too little time."

The first physicians to label this type of coronary-prone personality, Meyer Friedman, M.D., and Ray Rosenman, M.D., of San Francisco, wrote a book about it. Their book, *Type A Behavior and Your Heart*, popularized the definition of a "type A personality" in the 1970s. Their conclusion, based on a study, was that people who are time-conscious, competitive, impatient

4. Look at Your Risk Factors

waiting in lines or at other delays, often short-tempered, and prone to doing two things at once, such as reading while shaving, have the typical type A personality. In their study, they found that such people were more likely to develop coronary trouble than were people with more relaxed, "type B" personalities. They defined type B types as people who tend to put off work and decisions, seem to be under little time pressure, and are generally low-keyed. They also recognized that many of us combine type A and type B personality traits.

People with predominantly type A personalities have been the subject of more research in recent years. Some researchers have zeroed in on anger as the key factor in the greater risk of heart disease encountered by type A people. One study found that the angriest, least trusting, and most cynical subjects were 50 percent more likely to have coronary heart disease than people with more positive views of the world, and nearly six times more likely to suffer heart attacks. Other physicians believe that time urgency and compulsiveness may be as important as anger.

It is possible to change some of the basic components of type A personality to type B, many physicians believe, but it often requires professional help. Relaxation training, biofeedback techniques, meditation, tranquilizers, and sometimes psychotherapy can all help change or modify the harmful traits of type A behavior.

Not all physicians have accepted the type A personality theory, so its role as a risk factor is still controversial. But as with some of the other risk factors for which absolute proof is lacking, it seems to make good sense to attempt to eliminate it. Eliminating it probably can't harm you, and it may do you a lot of good in many ways. With a disease as serious as heart trouble, it behooves us to reduce risk factors rather than wait for absolute proof of their roles.

5.
Diagnosing Heart Problems

IF YOU HAVE heart disease today, you are much more fortunate than cardiac patients were only three decades ago. Thanks to a virtual revolution in diagnostic technology and knowledge, physicians are now able to detect and examine heart disease with a precision that was impossible in the past.

Until recent years, physicians trying to determine the causes and extent of heart trouble were handicapped by the fact that the heart is ordinarily invisible, hidden inside the rib cage. For more than a century, the most important diagnostic tool was the stethoscope. Still in use today, this sensitive listening instrument enables a doctor to hear a heart's beating much more clearly than it can be heard with the unaided ear. Through training and experience, a physician can distinguish certain sounds and rhythms associated with heart irregularities. For example, the sound of a normal heart is something like lub-dub. But a leaking heart valve makes a rasping sound, a too-thick valve a sharp click. As useful as a stethoscope is for detecting such abnormalities, however, it is not very useful in diagnosing many of the wide variety of things that can go wrong in the cardiovascular system.

THE ELECTROCARDIOGRAM

The other basic diagnostic tool physicians relied on in the past (and still use today) is the electrocardiogram (usually called an EKG, from the German spelling). This test records the heart's electrical activity, which can indicate a number of things about the heart's functioning. Up to a dozen electrodes are attached to a patient's chest, arms, and legs with suction cups. The wires connected to the electrodes lead to a recording machine, the electrocardiograph. A stylus, a kind of pen, records the changes in the heart's electrical activity as lines on special graph paper, in much the same way as the pen of a seismograph records earthquake activity, though the forms of energy are different. One cycle on the EKG reflects the electrical changes that occur during one complete heartbeat. The electrical charges are the same ones described in Chapter Two ("Nature's Marvelous Pump"), generated by nerve centers to make the heart contract and relax for most effective function. An experienced physician can learn much about the heart by studying the peaks and valleys on the electrocardiogram. If there are extra wiggles, or if the shape of a "peak" or "valley" differs from the shape recognized as normal, specific defects are indicated. The electrocardio-

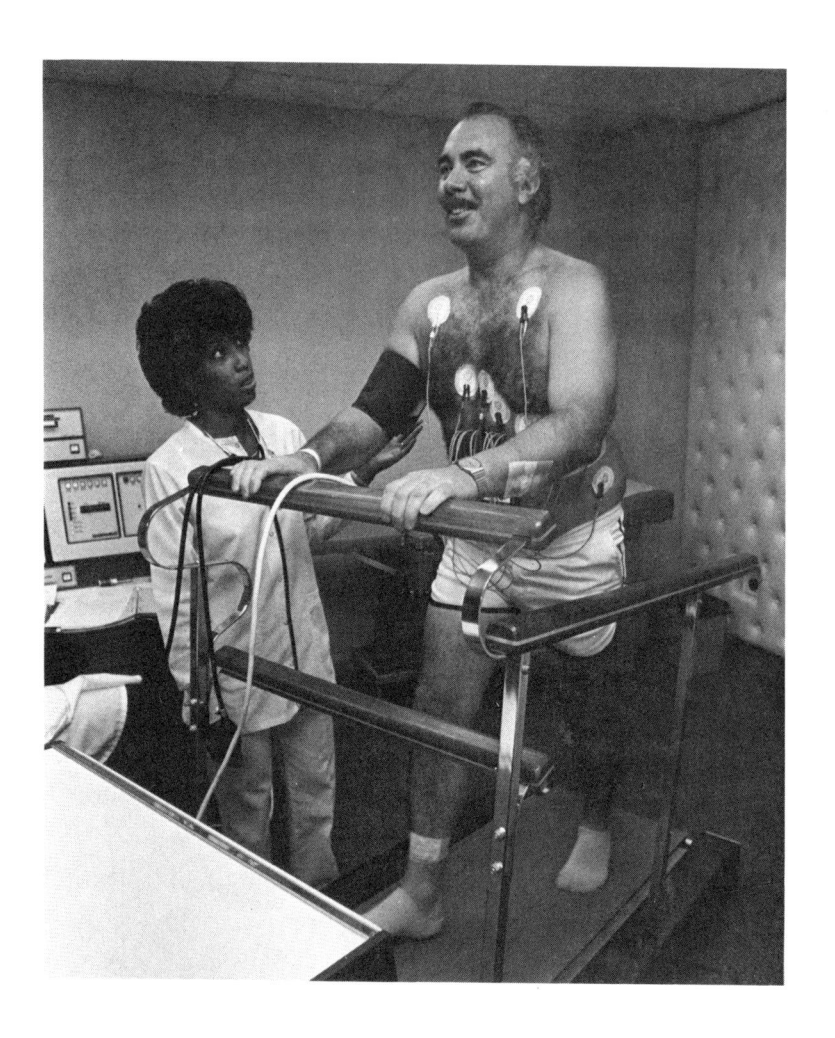

The electrocardiogram stress test, or exercise tolerance test, is a common diagnostic procedure. The strength of electrical impulses emitted by the heart during exercise is calibrated on graph paper. Heart muscle damage or impairment of adequate blood supply to the heart muscle (due to artery blockage) can often be identified by changes in the patterns of electrical impulses as the patient exercises and forces his heart to work harder. Both a physician and a nurse monitor the test procedure.

gram also precisely measures the heart rate, the number of beats per minute.

Unfortunately, the electrocardiogram is not foolproof. False readings may be obtained, because they usually are taken when the patient is resting, and a defective heart can appear to function normally when the body is resting, even though it functions abnormally when demands on it increase, as during exercise. Electrocardiograms are usually part of routine physical examinations, but if a physician knows of any symptoms associated with heart irregularities, he or she will want to conduct further, more specific tests.

Stress Tests

A common diagnostic procedure is the stress test (exercise tolerance test), which is used to measure the heart's electrical function during mild stress—the most likely time an abnormality would show up. A stress test can help to diagnose an inadequate supply of blood to the heart muscle (possibly caused by arterial blockage), disturbances in heart rhythm, or an impairment of heart muscle function. These abnormalities may not show up on a resting EKG.

Stress test patients are hooked up as in an EKG test, but with electrodes attached only to the chest, not the arms and legs, too. In some tests, the patient rides a stationary bicycle; in others, he or she walks on a motorized treadmill to obtain the required exercise. A target heart rate is determined in advance, based on the

5. Diagnosing Heart Problems

patient's age and general condition. In the treadmill test, the speed of the treadmill is increased at intervals, as is its incline. This is designed to make the patient work harder in stages, gradually increasing the heart rate up to the target rate. As the heart requires more and more oxygen (blood), the test may show that the blood supply to the heart is inadequate.

As a safety precaution, a doctor performs the test with a nurse or other medical personnel present. During the test, the blood pressure and the pulse rate are monitored to determine the effects of the exercise on the entire cardiovascular system. If the patient develops such symptoms as chest pain, or if the blood pressure or heart rates exceed predetermined levels of normalcy for the patient, the test is immediately terminated.

If the patient goes through the entire test (about ten minutes of exercise, depending on the patient's condition) without any indications of the heart not receiving enough blood as the requirement for blood is increased by exercise, the result is "negative." If there are indications that the heart is not receiving enough blood, the result is "positive."

The Thallium Stress Test

Even a stress EKG test may not always detect coronary artery disease. Another procedure, the thallium stress test, can sometimes show problems that might be missed on a regular stress EKG test. The thallium stress test is performed along with an EKG stress test, but it has an added feature. The patient still walks on a treadmill or rides a stationary bicycle to the predetermined peak point of exercise, but when that point is reached, a low-level radioactive substance or "dye" (thallium) is injected into the patient's arm. After the stress part of the test is completed, the patient lies on a special table or platform and a large nuclear scanning camera on a mechanical arm is placed over his or her chest. The patient lies there while the camera records the flow of thallium in the heart. The radiation emitted by the thallium is picked up by the camera and is then converted electronically into an image shown on a screen and in still pictures. Since the thallium collects in various parts of the heart muscle, the test can reveal changes that suggest that not enough blood (in which the thallium is carried) is reaching specific parts of the heart. Usually two thirty-minute scanning sessions are required in each test.

Holter Monitor

This portable EKG device is used to detect irregularities in heart rhythm in patients who may or may not have symptoms. Since the monitor is a small device that can be worn attached to a strap over the shoulder or around the waist, patients can wear it for 24 hours or even longer while they go about their normal routines. Electrodes are attached to the patient's chest in the manner of an EKG test and are connected to the Holter monitor. The patient keeps a diary during the test period, noting the times various activities were performed. This

5. Diagnosing Heart Problems

enables a physician to evaluate the heart's activity in relation to the physical activities during that time period.

ECHOCARDIOGRAM

Medical science has adapted the principles of sonar, used by ships to find submarines and other underwater objects and show their depth. The record is called an echocardiogram, which can provide accurate, detailed information about the inside of the heart, including the size of the heart's chambers, the functioning of the heart muscle, and the characteristics of the heart valves. It is also useful in documenting the presence of congenital heart disease.

The technique involves producing high-pitched (ultrasonic) sound waves that are inaudible to the human ear. These waves can be aimed and focused like light. They penetrate certain body tissues but are bounced back by the heart and blood vessels. Special equipment detects these echoes and converts them into an image of the heart's interior on a screen, while a small instrument like a microphone is passed repeatedly over the patient's chest. The medical technician using the instrument directs the sound pulse toward the heart, aiming away from the ribs and the lungs because they would produce extra reflections. The echoes bounce back from the heart, first from one exterior wall, then from internal structures, and finally from the opposite exterior wall. When converted by a computer into a screen image, the echoes reveal a cross section of the heart, its valves, internal structures, and blood flow.

PHONOCARDIOGRAM

In this test, an electronic sensor is used to detect and record heart sounds that are inaudible to the human ear and that may not be picked up by a stethoscope. One or more special microphones are attached to the patient's chest to pick up heart sounds. A recording machine creates a picture of the sound waves for a physician to interpret. Phonocardiogram tests are usually conducted in soundproof rooms because silence is required for the test to be valid. Used to supplement the EKG, phonocardiograms can help to detect restricted blood flow, an abnormal muscle contraction, and very early stages of heart valve disease.

THE CINE CORONARY ARTERIOGRAM

This important diagnostic procedure is the most accurate means yet developed to diagnose coronary artery disease and other heart ailments. It is often called the Gold Standard by which all other diagnostic tests are measured, because nothing else approaches its accuracy. Without it, there could not be open heart surgery.

Three decades ago, there was no diagnostic technique for pinpointing coronary artery disease. Unlike other heart ailments, coronary artery disease could not be heard with a stethoscope or recorded on an EKG. Many apparently healthy people had heart attacks or died before anyone realized that they were ill.

The conventional medical thinking at that time was that it was impossible to invade the arteries of the heart

5. Diagnosing Heart Problems

with a catheter and dyes to photograph the internal surfaces without causing death.

Then in 1958, F. Mason Sones, Jr., M.D., a cardiologist at the Cleveland Clinic Foundation, revolutionized the course of cardiology—proving that coronary visualization could be done, and should be done.

For the first time, doctors were able to see and photograph the arteries that carry life-sustaining blood to the heart muscle. They could accurately identify people suspected of having coronary disease but who actually had other ailments. And for patients with coronary artery disease, they now had a literal "road map" of the heart's blood supply, with the obstructions clearly visible.

Dr. Sones's technique, a linking of cardiac catheterization, fluoroscopy, and motion-picture making, is the most important advance in cardiology in this century. It is now standard throughout the world, providing the basis for assessing the value of surgery or other kinds of treatment. It makes the safe and effective repair of diseased hearts possible. And after open heart surgery, it can document the effectiveness of surgery in improving blood circulation.

"Without the work of Dr. Mason Sones—the most important contributor to modern cardiology—all our efforts in myocardial revascularization would have been fruitless," says noted cardiovascular surgeon Rene G. Favaloro, of Argentina, who was recognized as the pioneer of coronary bypass surgery for his work at the Cleveland Clinic Foundation in the 1960s. "Coronary

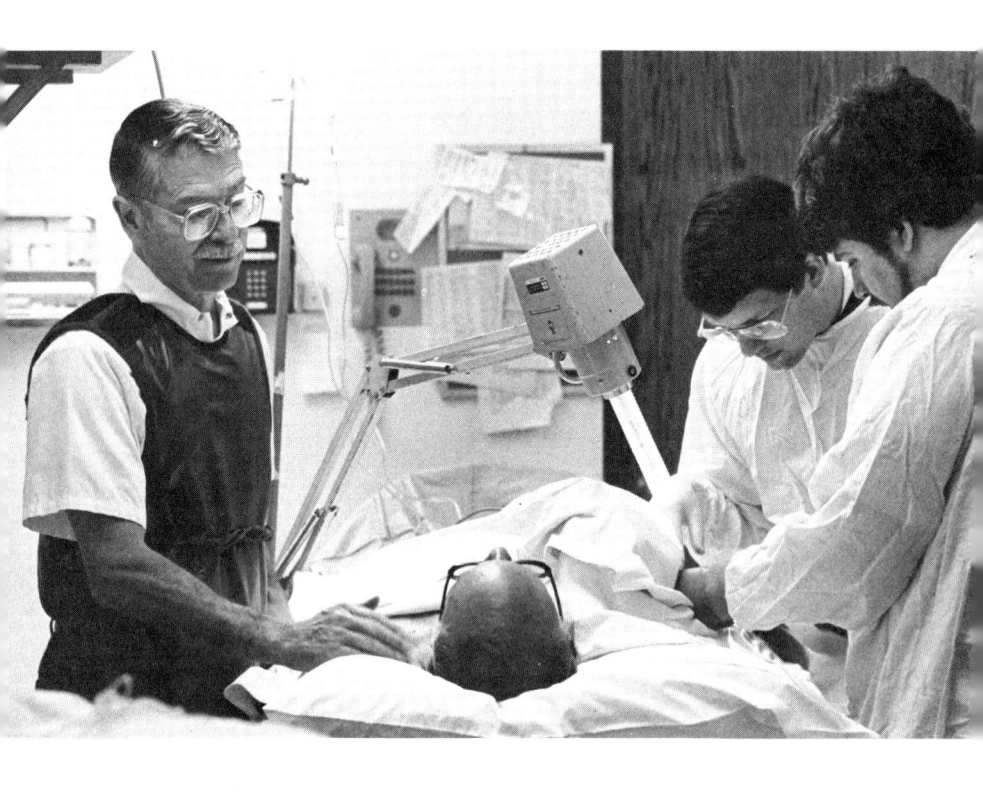

To obtain an angiogram, or "movie" of the coronary arteries, a physician threads a catheter through an artery to the patient's heart. The cardiologist in charge (*left*) is always assisted by one or more nurses or physicians. The patient remains awake during the cardiac catheterization procedure, which is used to locate coronary artery blockage.

5. Diagnosing Heart Problems

arteriography has become the Court of Last Appeal from which we learn the anatomy and even the physiology of coronary circulation."

A perfectionist, Dr. Sones was determined to perfect his technique and equipment. He taught himself the language of video engineering, the chemistry of dye compounds, the physics of optics and image amplification. He learned more about radiology than most radiologists knew. By teaching himself, he was able to communicate his needs to the engineers who designed the equipment he required.

Physicians from all over the world began sending their patients to Dr. Sones at the Cleveland Clinic Foundation for confirmation of their diagnoses and for validation of their attempts at surgical repair. Dr. Sones's findings were startling. One-third of the patients had been misdiagnosed. They had been living severely restricted lives, although there was nothing wrong with their hearts. And the surgical repairs Dr. Sones was seeing were often failures, as shown by his amazing films of arteries.

As quickly as Dr. Sones learned, he taught. Never greedy for accolades, he willingly shared what he knew with other doctors and medical personnel, and his teaching was so effective that many in the medical profession call the cardiology teams at the Cleveland Clinic the best in the world.

These coronary arteriograms became the blueprints for cardiovascular surgeons to work from. They proved the value of redirecting an internal mammary artery to bring blood directly into the heart muscle and also demonstrated the effectiveness of using the saphenous vein in the leg for bypass surgery grafts.

Hundreds of thousands of these arteriograms are performed every year in medical centers throughout the world. Though these tests may be considered common, they are not dismissed as routine procedures. They are invasive tests because a thin plastic tube (the catheter) is inserted into the patient's body. Although the procedure is virtually pain-free, requiring only a local anesthetic, it does carry a very slight risk of complications. Serious complications are rare (these are heart attacks, strokes, and death). Other complications include spasm of a coronary artery, which could damage the heart; an allergic reaction to the dye; and an abnormal heart rhythm.

Cine coronary arteriograms at most large medical centers are performed in special cardiac catheterization laboratories, which are well equipped. (At the Cleveland Clinic, four new state-of-the-art laboratories are named the Sones Laboratories in honor of the father of this procedure.) Cardiac catheterization is not considered surgery, but it is done under conditions as sterile as those in an operating room. Although some patients may be hospitalized before their catheterization, it is commonly done as an outpatient procedure.

A catheterization can be done from either the arm or the groin. The patient is awake during the procedure and can watch it on a television monitor. The doctor performing the test inserts a long, narrow, hollow tube into a blood vessel in an arm (brachial artery or vein) or the

5. Diagnosing Heart Problems

groin (femoral artery or vein) and guides it to the heart. The patient has EKG electrodes attached to his or her arms and legs to record the heart rhythm during the test. Inserting the catheter requires only a small incision after a local anesthetic has been applied. There is generally little discomfort.

The physician gradually threads the catheter through the blood vessels until the end of it passes through an artery to the heart. When the doctor is ready to look at the heart on the television screen, the lights will be dimmed. With the catheter in place, the doctor releases a small amount of a clear liquid contrast material (the dye) into the heart. As the heart beats, the dye outlines the arteries, valves, and heart chambers.

When the dye is injected into the left ventricle of the heart, the patient feels a hot flash for several seconds, which resembles the sensation when one stands in front of a just-opened oven door. Occasionally a patient feels nauseated, but this is not a common problem. In fact, there is very little discomfort, and the patient's eyes are often riveted to the television screen, where he or she can watch the catheter and the dye inside the beating heart.

A 35-millimeter motion picture camera with X-ray film is positioned directly over the table or cart on which the patient lies. The filming begins as soon as the dye is injected into the heart, and a complete movie is made showing the dye in the blood as it flows through the coronary arteries and the heart. The cardiologist performing the test needs to see as many different branches

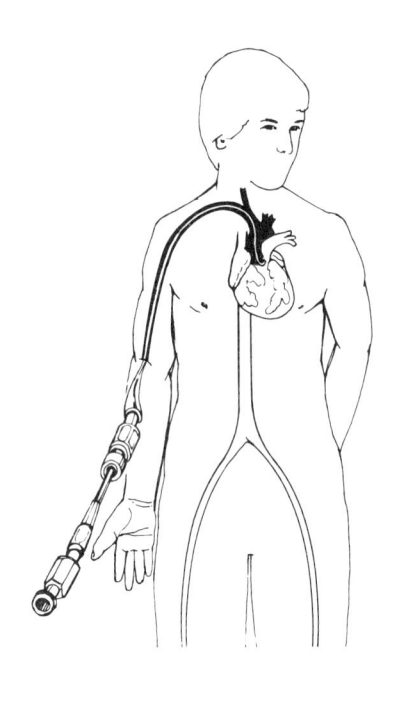

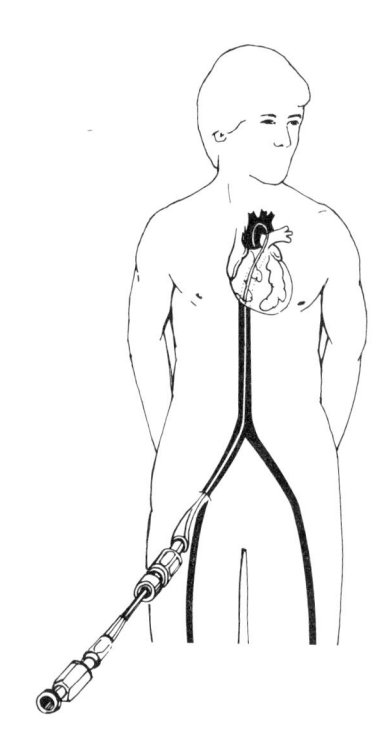

When cardiac catheterization is done through the arm (*left*), a small incision is made where the arm bends at the elbow, after a local anesthetic is applied. The catheter is inserted into an exposed blood vessel and threaded through vessels to the heart. It is then manipulated into the coronary arteries and heart chambers. A contrast material ("dye") is injected through the catheter so that X-ray movies may be taken of the vessels, chambers, and valves of the heart. In some cases the catheterization is done through the groin (*right*). After a local anesthetic is applied, an introducer sheath is used to puncture the skin— no incision is necessary. The catheter is passed through the sheath directly into the femoral artery and then to the heart. Both catheterization procedures are generally painless.

5. Diagnosing Heart Problems

of the arteries as possible, so filming is from several different views. The X-ray camera is rotated as more contrast material is injected.

When the filming is finished, the catheter is withdrawn from the body (this is not felt) and the small incision is closed with a few stitches. The procedure usually takes a little more than an hour. Patients who have the procedure performed from the leg are told to remain in bed for several hours after the test as a precaution, although generally there are no complications.

Cardiac catheterization, an expensive procedure, requires a specially trained cardiologist to perform it, and it can involve major as well as minor risks. For these reasons, it is not a test to be taken lightly, and doctors do not recommend it for everyone. But when a patient has symptoms, or when positive results have been obtained on such diagnostic tests as a stress EKG or a thallium stress test, it may be necessary to obtain more information. By observing the films, cardiologists and surgeons can determine where arteries are blocked and how bad the blockage is. No other test can give such precise information.

HARTFORD PUBLIC LIBRARY

6.
Should You Have Surgery?

TODAY's improved diagnostic tools and surgical procedures have made open heart surgery possible. There is no question that surgery, such as heart valve replacement and coronary bypasses (revascularization), has saved thousands of lives and improved the quality of life for great numbers of people with heart disease. But open heart surgery, particularly coronary bypass surgery, is such a recent development in the long history of medicine that doctors are still debating its usefulness for various types of patients. It has not been possible to measure the long-term effects of this surgery on heart disease, because less than twenty years have elapsed since its inception.

For most of medicine's history, physicians considered the heart untouchable. Hippocrates, regarded as the father of medicine, wrote, "A wound in the heart is mortal." Theodor Billroth, the famous Viennese surgeon who pioneered operations to remove stomach cancers, wrote in 1880, "Any surgeon who wishes to preserve the

6. Should You Have Surgery?

respect of his colleagues would never attempt to operate on the heart."

But emergency situations, such as knife and bullet wounds to the heart, when death was imminent, sometimes resulted in desperate surgical attempts to save lives, and by 1909, 109 cases of suturing of heart wounds had been described in the medical literature. About 60 percent of these patients did not survive, but without the surgery, the death rate would have been 100 percent. In the first half of this century, sporadic attempts were made to operate on the heart, but it had to be done almost blindly, on the beating heart. Without today's diagnostic tools, surgeons could not pinpoint the exact locations of heart ailments, so surgery was seldom attempted.

The dawn of the age of revascularization—the attempt to bring new blood vessels into the heart from another part of the body—came in 1932. It was then that Dr. Claude S. Beck of the Cleveland Clinic sutured a portion of the chest muscle to the surface of the heart to obtain more blood for the heart through the capillaries that developed between the two tissues. During the next fifteen years, a number of surgeons tried variations of this technique, grafting pieces of tissue from other nearby organs—the intestine, liver, and spleen—to obtain auxiliary sources of blood. Sometimes the operations seemed to work; sometimes they did not work. Without today's coronary angiography, surgeons could not see which coronary vessels were obstructed and could not tell which part of the heart had the insufficient blood supply. Later Dr. Beck tried to stimulate the flow of blood within the heart by irritating the surface of the heart muscle with such abrasives as talc and asbestos. The method was eventually discarded as one more earnest attempt in the long process of finding a surgical method of improving blood flow to the heart.

Shortly after World War II, a Canadian surgeon, Dr. Arthur M. Vineberg, tried implanting the open end of the left internal mammary artery into the heart muscle. He selected this artery because it is rarely afflicted with disease, it is not essential in the breast, and it is located near the heart. Dr. Vineberg believed that implanting the internal mammary artery into the heart muscle would stimulate small blood vessels in the heart to increase in size and link up to supply blood to part of the heart. He could not prove that this growth in "collateral" circulation occurred, however. Several years later, in 1958, the development of coronary angiography at the Cleveland Clinic Foundation allowed doctors there to examine the network of blood vessels in the heart. The new procedure confirmed the belief that tiny dormant vessels in the heart, the arterioles, gradually grow larger to receive and to distribute the new blood supply.

This type of operation had a major shortcoming, however. After the end of an internal mammary artery was implanted into the heart muscle, it took three to six months for the collateral vessels to grow sufficiently to increase the coronary blood circulation. Many heart patients could not survive that long without an improvement in their circulation. What was needed was a type of surgery that would increase the blood flow immediately.

6. Should You Have Surgery?

Vascular surgeons had been achieving this in the legs, where they cut out an entire segment of an obstructed artery and replaced it with an unclogged vein segment, but coronary arteries are much narrower and more difficult to work with.

Coronary angiography provided the breakthrough that made it possible to graft saphenous vein segments from the legs directly onto coronary arteries, creating bypasses around the obstructed segments of these arteries. Dr. Favaloro, who introduced this operation at the Cleveland Clinic Foundation, performed the first successful bypass surgery with a leg vein in 1967. He found that the saphenous vein in the leg was well suited for use in coronary bypass surgery because it was best able to withstand the high artery pressures without breaking or ballooning. Though the left internal mammary artery is even better in one respect—it tends to remain unclogged longer after bypass surgery—there are only two such arteries. So the saphenous vein graft is the most common bypass procedure, since multiple bypasses are usually necessary.

Between 1967 and 1970, Dr. Favaloro and his fellow staff members performed 1,310 bypass grafts, perfecting the techniques of the operation. Nearly 90 percent of these early patients were able to resume their normal activities and were free of debilitating angina. Surgeons at other medical institutions soon undertook the new surgical procedure; and coronary bypass surgery today is now a common operation, performed at medical institutions throughout the United States and in many other countries.

But who should have bypass surgery? This is where members of the medical profession disagree. Although there is a near-unanimous agreement among medical professionals that coronary bypass surgery usually eliminates angina and enhances the quality of life for patients, the question of whether it prolongs life is still being studied and debated, as discussed earlier.

Rather than one simple answer, there are a variety of answers that depend on the location and severity of the patient's coronary artery disease. For example, virtually all the studies conducted to date indicate that patients with obstructions of the left main coronary artery, often a life-threatening condition, live longer after bypass surgery than those who forgo surgery in favor of drug therapy. And the results of a national study released in the past year show similar advantages of surgery for patients with obstructions in all three principal coronary arteries. The Veterans Administration conducted a nine-year study of about 800 cardiac patients, half of whom underwent bypass surgery while the other half had drug therapy. The surgery patients had obstructions of the three main coronary arteries plus abnormalities of the left ventricle, the heart's main pumping chamber. The VA Cooperative Study, conducted at VA hospitals throughout the United States, showed a 40 percent increase in the survival rate of triple bypass patients over patients who did not have surgery. An analysis of survival rates during a nine-year follow-up study showed that 70 percent of the patients undergoing triple bypass

6. Should You Have Surgery?

operations were still alive, compared with only 51 percent of those patients who did not have the surgery.

The VA study results support the recent findings from the European Coronary Surgery Trial, a similar study showing that, after eight years, 94 percent of the patients who had bypass surgery were still alive, compared with 82 percent of those patients treated only with drugs.

The Cleveland Clinic Foundation keeps careful records on its bypass surgery patients and monitors them continuously. By studying the first 1,000 of its bypass patients each year, Foundation physicians have confirmed that people with left main artery disease and three-vessel disease do better with surgery than without. Five years after their surgery, 91 percent of these patients are still alive, and that figure is rising despite the growing number of difficult cases referred to the Cleveland Clinic. Without surgery, only about 57 percent of those patients would have survived. And these figures do not take into account the fact that many of the patients who die within five years do so from causes unrelated to coronary artery disease or to their surgery.

At least one study, however, has indicated different results for other patients—patients with mild to moderate chest pain with blockages in one or more arteries and patients with no chest pain, who have had a heart attack. The National Heart, Lung and Blood Institute financed a ten-year study of patients at fifteen medical centers; the results of this study were announced in 1984. The study was conducted among 780 patients who were randomly assigned to be treated either with surgery or drugs. At the end of six years, 92 percent of those who had surgery and 90 percent of those treated only with drugs were still alive, a difference that is not statistically significant.

The physicians who directed the study suggested that patients who have milder symptoms of coronary artery disease might be better off postponing bypass surgery until their symptoms worsen. "We now know that it is safe to wait to operate if and when the patient's symptoms get significantly worse," said Eugene Passamani, M.D., associate director of cardiology at the National Heart, Lung and Blood Institute. "The next stage of mild angina is usually not a heart attack or sudden death but rather a worsening of the angina.

"In fact," Dr. Passamani continued, "it may be safer in the long run to wait, since bypass surgery does not cure the underlying disease, which usually progresses even after a bypass operation." Ten years after surgery, the study indicated, the grafted vessels are also obstructed in 40 percent of the patients. And half of the remaining 60 percent of the patients develop further significant narrowing of coronary arteries.

Many patients with more narrowing of their coronary arteries undergo a second bypass operation to relieve progression of their disease. "But repeat surgery is technically more difficult because of scar tissue and carries higher risk with less symptomatic relief than the first operation," according to Dr. Passamani, "so it may pay to wait until that first operation is really needed if the patient has only mild angina."

6. Should You Have Surgery?

Physicians at leading centers for the treatment of cardiovascular disease recognize these different categories of patients being considered for surgery. Patients with left main artery disease and triple vessel disease are the most likely candidates for bypass surgery. Those with less blockage and less serious symptoms should be evaluated on an individual basis.

"At the Cleveland Clinic Foundation, we feel strongly that the decision on coronary bypass surgery must be made on an individual basis," says William P. Sheldon, M.D., chairman of the Department of Cardiology. "After studying all the aspects of a patient's condition, we have to decide when that patient's disease is life-threatening and can be treated through surgery."

The patient's angiograms are reviewed jointly by cardiologists and cardiovascular surgeons at the Cleveland Clinic, and together they reach a decision on whether the patient would benefit from surgery. Their decisions are backed by an ongoing study that began at the Foundation in the early days of cardiac catheterization. William L. Proudfit, M.D., then chairman of Clinical Cardiology, studied the records of patients undergoing the procedure. Dr. Proudfit followed the natural course of coronary artery disease in those who were treated medically. He established that the location and severity of the obstructions in the coronary arteries, coupled with how well the heart muscle works, will predict someone's likelihood of death without surgery. From this and other studies, the need for a permanent registry became apparent. What began as a card file is today the largest, most compre-

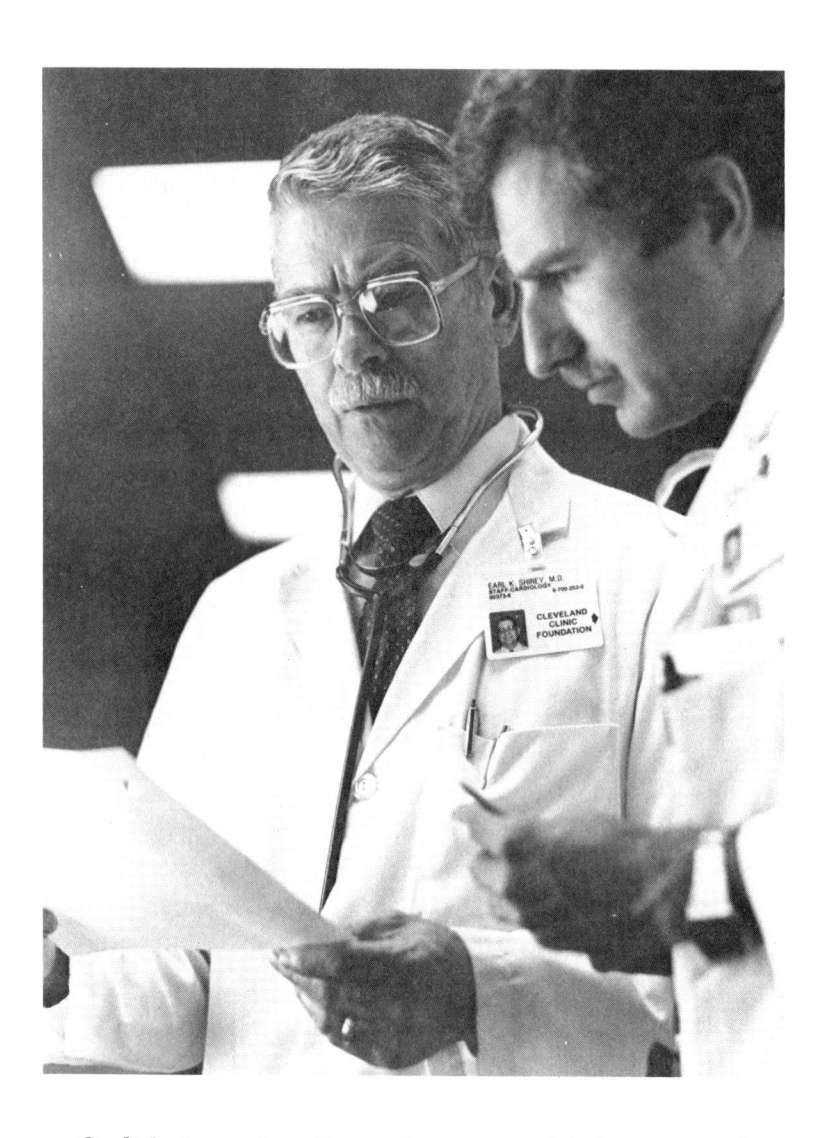

Cardiologists and cardiovascular surgeons jointly review each patient's angiograms and other clinical data at the Cleveland Clinic to reach decisions on whether or not the patient would benefit from open heart surgery. Not every patient would benefit from surgery, and the doctors' recommendations must be determined on an individual, case-by-case basis.

6. Should You Have Surgery?

hensive computerized cardiovascular registry in the world.

The continual evaluation of patients' conditions and how successful their treatment is over time allows Foundation physicians to provide the most effective course of therapy. "The choice is rarely medicine versus surgery," says Dr. Sheldon. "The answer usually lies between [them], in the best combination of medical and interventional therapies for each patient. This may include drugs, a change of life-style, angioplasty (balloon catheterization to reduce obstructions) and/or surgery."

Dr. Shirey of the Cleveland Clinic has pointed out that the decision for or against bypass surgery is a complicated one, taking into account many factors in each patient's case. "Surgery is not a panacea; it plays a role in selected cases," he says. "In selecting patients for surgery, it's important to do a very careful examination in terms of the patient's history and physical examination. In some cases it's necessary to conduct stress tests. And it's mandatory before selecting a patient for surgery to conduct a coronary angiogram. We must take into account the symptoms, the degree of blockage in the arteries, and the number of arteries that are obstructed. In the angiograms we look for the presence or absence of collateral vessels—spontaneous bypasses that have developed as a result of the blockages. We observe how well the patient responds to medication. As we look at each obstructed artery, we have to determine how important that vessel is to the heart, how much heart muscle is being supplied by that vessel, and what may happen if that vessel becomes completely obstructed."

A patient facing the prospect of bypass surgery is naturally concerned about the risk of death during the operation. The statistics should be reassuring. More than one million people have had coronary bypass surgery since the operation was developed, and the fatality rates are very low. A national study gave it as 1.3 percent at leading medical centers. The rate is even lower at the Cleveland Clinic Foundation—less than 1 percent. However, the death rate is higher for this surgery at some smaller hospitals where fewer bypass operations are performed. Experts in this field say that a cardiovascular surgeon has to perform a minimum of three bypass operations a week to keep his proficiency at an acceptable level, and this might not be the case at some smaller institutions. Any patient considering such surgery at any medical institution is justified in inquiring about the number of operations performed.

It should also be noted that not all bypass operations are successful. Some national studies have shown that between 10 and 20 percent of the bypass vessels grafted to the arteries become blocked within the first year after surgery. After that, the studies show that about 2 percent per year become blocked. But the odds are still good that an operation will be successful.

Nearly all the studies show that bypass surgery usually improves a patient's life. Almost every study conducted to date has shown that bypass surgery patients have less

6. Should You Have Surgery?

pain from angina, need less medication, and can exercise more than patients treated medically.

Dr. Delos Cosgrove, who has performed thousands of coronary bypass operations at the Cleveland Clinic Foundation, says, "Bypass surgery is the only form of therapy that can increase the life expectancy of patients with severe coronary artery disease. But just as important is the fact that after surgery these patients feel good again and are optimistic about the future. They have energy to resume work, volunteer activities and family duties. Their quality of life improves tremendously. Bypass surgery can make the difference between living and just existing."

7.
Preparing for Surgery

ONCE YOU HAVE decided to undergo open heart surgery, after consulting with your physician, your family, and perhaps getting a second opinion from another physician, there is usually some sense of relief that the decision has been made and the uncertainty ended. But with the realization that you are actually going to have the operation come anxiety and apprehension. This is to be expected, of course—it has been said that nobody ever walked into a hospital without some apprehension, unless he worked there. A hospital is a strange, foreign environment to most of us, and we don't like to think about it. We know we're going to have a fearful experience, and we don't know much about what will take place.

Fear of the unknown is a common human experience, and the best way to reduce or eliminate the fear is to learn and understand. In the case of impending surgery, the best way to reduce apprehension is to find out what

7. Preparing for Surgery

to expect in the hospital. A patient can do this by asking his or her doctor as many questions as possible (jotting down a list of questions is a good idea before meeting with the doctor). Many hospitals have brochures that answer many questions, and books such as this one serve the purpose of educating patients about heart disease and heart surgery. The more you learn about what is going to happen in the hospital, the less anxiety you will have.

At most hospitals, patients are admitted two or three days before the surgery is scheduled. This time is used by the hospital staff to conduct the routine preoperative tests. At the Cleveland Clinic Foundation, an innovative program, established in 1981, permits patients who are not at immediate risk to come in as outpatients for tests and instructions in advance of the surgery date. Then they can go home and not be admitted to the hospital until the day before their surgery is scheduled. The purpose of the program, called TCI ("to come in") is to reduce the costs and inconveniences of surgery. Today about one-half of the Foundation's patients qualify for the TCI program, which saves them an average of 11 percent of their hospital bill. This is no small consideration for both the patients and their insurance companies. It has been estimated that the national average of total costs for a coronary bypass operation is about $25,000.

For patients entering the Cleveland Clinic the traditional way, the routine goes something like this: Two days before your surgery date, you usually are admitted in the afternoon or evening, at an assigned time. The first stop is the admitting office, where you fill out admitting forms. You should bring pertinent insurance information, such as your Blue Cross, Blue Shield insurance card. (You also should have your personal toilet articles and a bathrobe and slippers, if you prefer these to the garb provided by the hospital.)

Once the forms have been filled out, you are escorted through a maze of hallways and elevators to your room on a nursing floor. You will be welcomed by a nurse from this unit, who will explain the hospital routine and take your temperature and blood pressure, and determine your pulse and respiration rate, procedures that will be repeated many times during your stay. At some point after you get comfortable and perhaps turn on your television set, you will be visited and checked by one or more staff physicians from the Cardiology Department.

At another point early in your stay, a staff person will take blood samples. Most of us have had blood samples taken at some time in our lives, and though it isn't a particularly pleasant experience, it isn't an excruciatingly painful one, either. The laboratory technician or nurse inserts a fine needle into a vein in your arm and withdraws a small amount of blood into test tubes. The laboratory will process these samples so your blood can be typed and cross-matched. Then if you need additional blood during surgery or afterward, the staff will know the type you need. Blood samples have other uses, too: red and white corpuscle counts can be taken, blood sugar and cholesterol levels can be measured, and the function of your liver, kidneys, and some endocrine glands can be evaluated.

7. Preparing for Surgery

The next day you are sent to the spirometry area, where a pulmonary or inhalation therapist measures your breathing capacity. You are asked to take a deep breath and blow as hard as you can into a plastic tube connected to a machine. This machine measures the force with which you exhale. Then you have a chest X-ray, a common procedure in which you stand with your chest against a large, opaque "window" that contains film and hold your breath while you are X-rayed. After this, you lie on an examining table in another department and have an electrocardiogram taken—another routine procedure most of us are familiar with. You are visited by your cardiologist on the Clinic staff, which provides a good opportunity for you to ask questions about the operation, the recovery routine, or anything else you want to know. Your surgeon or his assistant will also visit you.

Not long after all the testing and interviewing are completed, you find you are being sent to "school" in the afternoon. Your first "class" is about breathing, which may surprise you, since it's something you've been doing without instructions your whole life. But breathing properly and coughing are going to be very important after this operation. In this class, conducted by an inhalation therapist, you learn why it is important to breath deeply and cough to clear your lungs. During the surgery and afterward, the lungs tend to retain fluids, which must be eliminated to avoid pneumonia. You and your classmates are given a clear, vertical plastic tube with a hose and mouthpiece attached. As you inhale, a little ball in the tube rises toward the top of the tube. The longer and

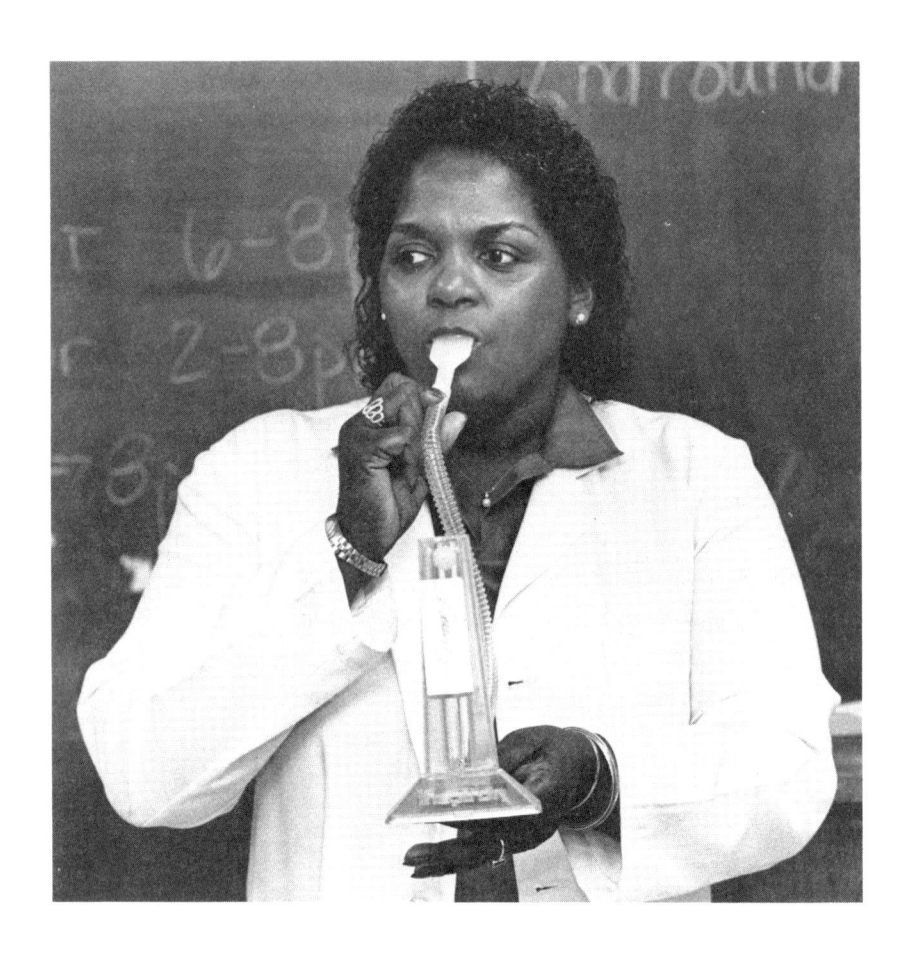

A day or so before open heart surgery, patients are instructed by an inhalation therapist about the importance of breathing deeply and coughing to clear their lungs of fluid during postoperative recovery. Each patient is given a plastic inhalation device to use every two hours during recuperation. The device helps to demonstrate the strength and duration of inhalation and encourages the patient to take deep breaths repeatedly.

7. Preparing for Surgery

more vigorously you can inhale, the higher the ball rises and the longer it stays up. The therapist tells you to inhale and push the ball toward the top, and to keep inhaling as long as you can so that the ball stays up while you time yourself. Your best time is recorded; there will be a variation in the performance of individuals in the class. Whereas some patients can keep the ball up for as long as fifteen seconds, others can keep it up for only two seconds.

This "toy" is yours to keep, and you are asked to take it with you to your room and to practice with it. You will be using it every two hours in the days after your operation, as a means of forcing yourself to breath deeply. You will be requested to take two or three breaths, using the toy, and then to cough as deeply as you can while sitting upright. This helps to clear your lungs of fluid. A therapist or nurse usually is there to help expel fluids and phlegm by pounding on your back while you cough.

It is painful to cough after the operation, at least at first, because your breastbone has been sliced down the middle and then wired back together again. The first time you are asked to cough, you'll feel as though your chest is in danger of splitting open—which, of course, it is not. The nurses recommend that you hold a pillow tightly to your chest as you cough, because it makes you feel better about your chest staying intact. And it does reduce the pain.

Emerging from the breathing and coughing class, you find yourself scheduled for yet another class. You are invited to bring your spouse or some other member of your family to this class, where a staff member will explain in detail what will happen during your surgery and recovery period. The staff member tells your relatives how to be kept informed of your progress, how to obtain information, where to wait during the operation, and so on. Your family is also given a telephone number to call if they go home. And they are told to leave a number where they can be reached.

Heart patients can also attend a diet class. A nutritionist discusses foods that are low in salt, and the use of salt substitutes, to reduce sodium in your diet and thus help to control hypertension. He or she also tells you how to avoid saturated fats (found in meat and dairy products and in certain prepared foods) and answers questions about cholesterol levels and the possible role of cholesterol in atherosclerosis.

Many patients and their relatives find it difficult to comprehend or retain much of what they are told in some of these classes before surgery. That is why it's sometimes a good idea to wait and attend the nutrition classes several days after the operation. The Cleveland Clinic and many other large hospitals have specially trained counselors to help patients and their families. The counselor, usually a nurse, can answer a great many questions about what will happen during and after the operation. This person is trained to look for emotional stress in patients and families and to try to alleviate it by being understanding and helpful.

Having a counselor present when a surgeon or cardiologist tells the patient about the impending surgery can

7. Preparing for Surgery

be helpful, because the patient may be so anxious that he or she doesn't hear everything the doctor says. The counselor can answer many of the patient's or the family's questions later and help them to interpret the information.

Danni Gogol Nadler, R.N., cardiovascular counselor at the Cleveland Clinic Foundation, explained her role thus: "The counselor's presence is important in order to increase the patient's and family's sense of security and to reduce feelings of panic and frustration. The counselor becomes a trusted friend who can answer questions and provide a helping hand for coming to grips with the situation.

"When patients or their families feel threatened and fearful, anything that is said or done may heighten these fears. Because patients and families come to the hospital with varying degrees of knowledge, understanding, and acceptance of heart disease, interpretation of the patient's condition may differ from one member to another. It is important, therefore, to determine as quickly as possible the extent of their understanding, so that an ongoing process of improving their knowledge can be instituted. Cardiovascular counseling is not only concerned with the immediate crisis situation but must also help the patient resolve the long-term implications of a chronic disease.

"The purpose, therefore, of counseling is to help each family member perceive the illness in such a way that they will be emotionally ready to move on to a better understanding and acceptance of the future, so that they can enjoy optimal health and well-being."

The evening before your operation, you are given an ordinary meal (it will be low in fat) and you can visit with your family in your room. However, the visiting will be interrupted somewhat by an orderly who will shave off most of the hair on your body while you talk through a privacy curtain. The shave is important because it not only provides a sterile operative area, it also will make it much less painful to remove adhesive bandages later.

You will also be requested to shower, but with a special antibacterial soap.

You may be given a light snack of juice and crackers, or something similar, before 10:00 P.M. But you will be instructed that after that, nothing except a sip of water may be taken by mouth. Patients should not have partially digested foods in their stomachs when they undergo surgery.

The last thing you will take by mouth will be a sedative to relax you and to help you sleep soundly through the night. This is a blessing, because it prevents you from tossing, turning, and worrying on the eve of this major event.

This is the preoperative routine at the Cleveland Clinic. It is similar to what you will experience at many large hospitals where open heart surgery is performed— a carefully planned set of procedures designed to accomplish the necessary preparation while making the patient and his or her family as comfortable as possible.

8.

Open Heart Surgery

When you awake the morning of the day of your surgery, you may have only a short waiting period, if your operation is scheduled for morning, or half the day if it is scheduled for afternoon. In any case, you will have some time to visit with your spouse or other relatives. You may be given a tranquilizer to alleviate the jitters. This is the time to give your personal possessions to your relatives to take home and to turn over to your nurse the things you will want later in your room but won't use in the recovery room or the intensive care unit. They will be stored for safekeeping.

Finally the appointed time arrives, and two orderlies enter your room with a cart or bed on wheels. You climb onto this and slide under a sheet, wearing only the ubiquitous hospital gown issued you. Your relatives can say good-bye to you here, or they can walk beside the cart as far as the elevator. Emotionally this parting is harder on your family than it is on you, thanks to the tranquilizer you have been given an hour earlier. Your mood most likely will be one of accepting what is to come, while your spouse or other relatives will be fearful and anxious. They will be directed to the family waiting lounge where they can read educational material about the surgery and, later, talk with your surgeon about the outcome of the operation.

Procedures for open heart surgery are similar at most large hospitals. Here is how a typical operation goes at the Cleveland Clinic:

The patient is wheeled to the surgical unit and into a "prep" area, the induction room. Still conscious but usually a little drowsy, the patient is prepared here for the monitoring of vital body functions during the operation. Catheters are inserted to aid in obtaining information. One catheter, at the wrist, will serve to measure blood pressure. Another is inserted into an arm vein to act as the conduit for the anesthetic. The central venous pressure line is inserted at the bend of an elbow and threaded into the vena cava, the large vein leading to the heart. It will be used to measure venous blood pressure and also to inject medication or blood almost directly into the heart very quickly. Another catheter is inserted into the pulmonary artery to measure pressure in that artery and help to evaluate heart performance. Sometimes another catheter is inserted into the jugular vein in the neck. Electrodes are attached on both sides of the upper body and will be connected to an electrocardiograph. None of this is painful to the patient, because

8. Open Heart Surgery

after the initial pinprick of the anesthesia catheter, the anesthetic takes effect.

When brought into the operating room, most patients are still awake, but are very groggy. If sufficiently awake to look around, patients at the Cleveland Clinic may be surprised to see that the operating room is not some big amphitheater, but a rather ordinary-looking room of no great size. You will also find it very chilly because you are lying naked under a sheet. To reduce the growth of bacteria and germs, operating rooms are kept at temperatures in the low sixties. The air pressure in these rooms is kept slightly higher than that in the hallways outside the doors so that the air in the room is forced out and the outside air, which contains bacteria, cannot flow into the room.

The room is crammed with the equipment needed for open heart surgery and the members of the surgical team are bustling around. The operating table is at the center, under high-intensity, adjustable overhead lights. At the foot of the operating table is the instrument table, with all the "tools" neatly arranged and sterilized, ready to be handed to the surgeon by the scrub nurse. Another table, also within easy reach, holds dressing, bandages, and the large gauze pads called sponges that are used during surgery.

Also nearby, for convenient viewing by the surgeon and his assistants, is some space-age-appearing equipment, the physiological data monitor, a collection of several television screens and digital readout devices.

The catheters and electrodes connecting the patient's body to this equipment make it possible to view the heart's electrical activity (EKG), arterial blood pressure, venous pressure, temperature, and so on. Another sophisticated, and vital, piece of equipment is the heart-lung machine, which will take over the function of the heart and lungs during surgery.

Teamwork is the key to the Cleveland Clinic's world-famous expertise at open heart surgery, and a well-drilled, experienced surgical team performs each operation. On an average day at the Clinic, eight eleven-member teams perform about fifteen operations—80 percent of them coronary bypass procedures. The surgeon in command of the team usually has at least one, and often two, physicians who are doing their residencies in cardiac surgery to assist him. In addition, there are cardiovascular nurse clinicians, scrub nurses, circulating nurses, anesthesia physicians (anesthesiologists) and nurses, and a cardiovascular perfusionist. All these professionals are specially trained in cardiac surgery. Also there are often surgeons from other hospitals who come to observe the operations and learn the Cleveland Clinic's techniques.

The scrub nurse, so-called because she must do the preoperative "scrub"—a timed washing of her hands and forearms with a special antiseptic solution—like the surgeons, comes into direct contact with the patient and handles the surgical instruments. The scrub nurse hands the surgical instruments and sterile equipment to the surgeon as he requests them during the operation. Having

8. Open Heart Surgery

set up the instrument and sponge and bandage tables before the operation, she has the responsibility, along with the circulating nurse, to count every instrument and sponge or bandage at the end of the surgery. These must be counted at least twice before the incision is closed, to ensure that nothing is left inside the patient.

The circulating nurse acts as a sort of manager of the operating room environment, being generally responsible for everything but the operation itself. She is called a circulating nurse because she circulates in and out of the operating room, getting supplies, bringing specimens to the laboratory for analysis, and so on. Her job is to see that conditions are right for the surgical team—the temperature, lights, electrical system, and supplies must be constantly monitored. Each detail of the operation is written down on forms, so that a permanent record is available. The circulating nurse does this, too.

The anesthesiologist team performs a vital role in any operation, including open heart surgery. The anesthesiologist is responsible for making sure that the unconscious patient is in good condition during and after surgery. This professional is busy throughout the operation, constantly monitoring such vital signs as blood circulation, breathing patterns, and heart activity. In coordination with the surgeon, the anesthesiologist administers drugs and fluids to maintain body functions at optimal levels, making adjustments as necessary. He or she continues to regulate these body functions until the end of the operation, when a procedure that returns the body to its natural state is followed.

Perfusionists, who operate the heart-lung machine, also have a vital responsibility. During the part of the operation when the heart is stilled so the surgeon can work on it, this machine is the only thing keeping the patient alive. The perfusionist sets up the machine before each operation, threading yards of tubing through the pumps, testing its operation, and making sure it will operate when needed. The perfusionist controls and adjusts the pressure and flow of the blood as it is circulated through the machine and back to the patient's body. He or she monitors the vital signs of the patient and reports them to the surgeon when requested.

These are the people the groggy patient sees as they busy themselves connecting him or her to the monitors and otherwise preparing for surgery. The surgeon himself may only appear briefly to greet the patient, because he is usually busy doing other things. He reviews the angiograms of each patient with a cardiologist just before the operation, stepping into a small, darkened booth to view the ghostly films he and the cardiologist can read so expertly, to pinpoint the areas of coronary artery obstruction.

"You'll be going to sleep very soon now," the anesthesiologist tells the patient, and this is usually the last thing the patient hears until the operation is over. The anesthesiologist has a number of anesthetics to choose from, and selects the ones best suited to the patient at hand. These put a patient to sleep very quickly, and paralyze the muscles as well. Some of them have an

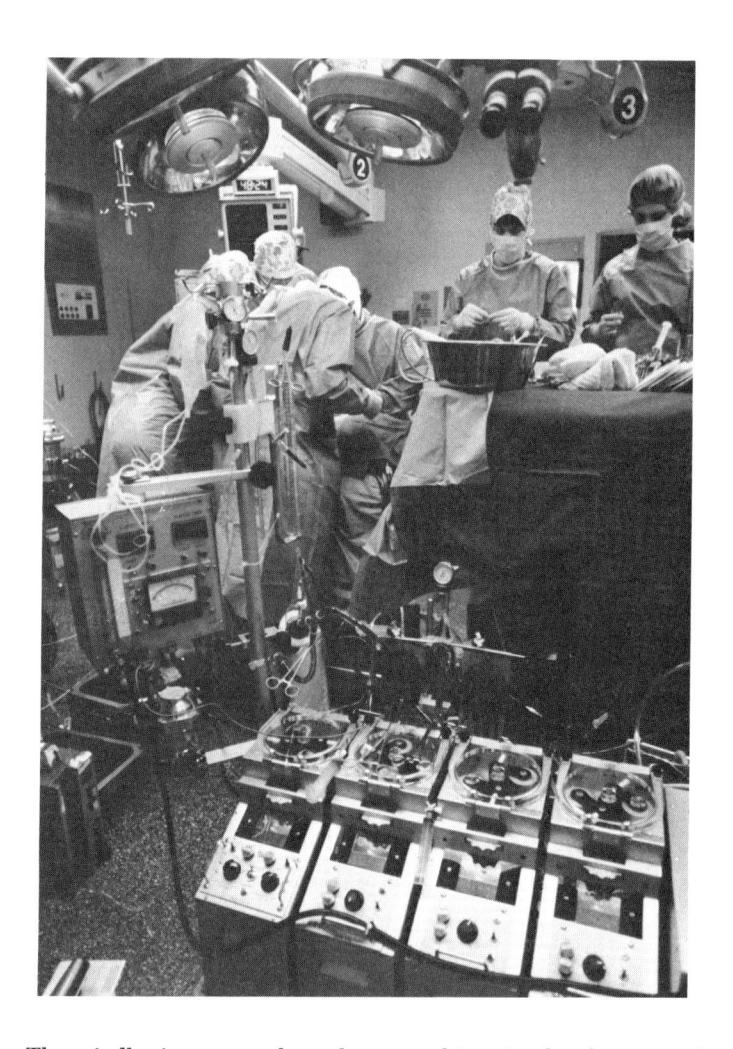

The vitally important heart-lung machine in the foreground makes it possible to stop the patient's heart from beating while surgery is performed on it. As the blood circulates continuously, the oxygen-depleted blood travels from the patient through the machine, where it is enriched with oxygen and sheds carbon dioxide; it then returns to travel throughout the body. Thus the machine performs the same functions normally provided by the heart and lungs, sometimes for several hours.

PATASKALA PUBLIC LIBRARY
101 SOUTH VINE STREET
PATASKALA, OHIO 43062

amnesic effect, and this is why many patients don't remember much about the first twenty-four hours in the recovery room after the operation. The patient's breathing and other vital functions are maintained by the equipment in the operating room.

The anesthesiologist pulls the unconscious patient's head back and inserts a device, the laryngoscope, down his or her throat to straighten the airway. An endotracheal tube about one-half an inch wide is slipped down the throat past the vocal cords. A balloon at the lower end of the tube is inflated to secure the tube and to make an airtight seal. The anesthesiologist pumps the mechanically operated air bag, which does the patient's breathing, and listens to the chest with a stethoscope to make sure the tube is in position and the apparatus is working. A smaller tube is inserted through the patient's nose and slipped down to the stomach to serve as a vent for digestive fluids and gases. The eyes are taped shut to keep them from drying out. A catheter is inserted into the bladder to collect urine, and a temperature probe is inserted in the rectum.

Next a nurse paints the patient's torso and legs with a yellow antiseptic, Betadine. The patient is covered with sterile green cotton cloth, which leaves exposed only the areas where the surgery will be done—the chest and the leg from which the saphenous veins will be taken. This cloth even covers a small frame over the patient's head, so that only the anesthesiologist, who stands at the head of the operating table, can see it.

8. Open Heart Surgery

Surgery now begins, not by the surgeon, but by one of his surgical residents. The resident examines the leg for the pattern of the saphenous vein that runs down the inside, sometimes tracing it with a felt-tipped pen. Working with his assistant, the surgical resident makes four incisions along the path of the vein, from the upper thigh down to the calf. They need to "harvest" this vein by digging deep into the flesh, cutting the vein free from the tissue surrounding it. Bleeding is kept to a minimum by the use of electrical cauteries, which resemble soldering irons and which instantly seal off the tributary veins. Usually the surgical resident leaves the rest of the job to his assistant, who requires about an hour to remove a long segment of the vein (a foot or more) and to tie off the ends of the vein that are left inside the leg. The assistant places the long segment of vein on a sterile cloth, carefully inspects it for tears, and staples its branch holes closed. He next tests the vein for leaks by injecting one end of it with a saline solution from a syringe. When he's satisfied that the vein is suitable for grafting, he places it in a container until the surgeon is ready to use it. The surgeon may test and examine the vein himself before using it. The leg can do without this saphenous vein segment, since there are many other vessels in the leg to carry blood.

Meanwhile the surgical resident has moved to the patient's chest. Using a curved surgical blade, he makes a shallow incision down the middle of the chest from the base of the neck. The blood behind the blade makes only a thin red line before the bleeding is stopped by cauterization. Now he slices more deeply, through a layer of yellowish fat. Again bleeding is controlled by cauterizing the tiny vessels. At last the breastbone is visible in the incision, showing pure white under the lights.

Now comes the most dramatic incision in an open heart operation—one that a squeamish layman would not choose to watch, but one that is performed with an impressive sure-handedness and expertise. The surgical resident is handed a small surgical saw, something like a jigsaw. Starting at the top of the incision, near the base of the neck, he inserts the blade and, while holding the saw with both hands, deftly pulls it down the middle of the breastbone, splitting the bone as neatly as a piece of wood. He and an assistant pull the two sets of ribs apart at the middle with their hands so they can insert a metal device, a retractor, in the middle of the cavity. When the resident turns a crank on the U-shaped retractor, the two sides of the rib cage swing open at the center, like the halves of a drawbridge opening toward the sky. This creates a surgical field, or area, to operate on, one about nine inches long by six inches wide. In the middle of this deep cavity the pericardium, the shining sac that encloses the heart, can be seen.

The operation has reached the crucial stage, repairing the heart itself. In a coronary bypass operation—let's say, a typical triple bypass procedure—this is when the staff cardiac surgeon enters. Up to this point, the members of the surgical team have gone about their work in a businesslike manner, chatting amiably as they work.

8. Open Heart Surgery

Often, there is soft background music playing to create a more pleasant, less nerve-wracking atmosphere. But when the surgeon, the commander of the team, enters the room, there is a certain amount of tension. The absolute boss, his orders are law, and woe betide the team member who fails to perform a duty to the surgeon's satisfaction. He is likely to be very demanding, a perfectionist who insists that every procedure meets his own high standards.

Surgeons, when they are working in operating rooms, know they must exercise authority in a way that keeps every member of the team on his toes. Since there is no room for carelessness, some surgeons deliberately foster an operating-room atmosphere in which every team member is alert and ready to respond instantly to orders. Some surgeons like to have background music playing; others forbid it. Some will engage in a certain amount of small talk or banter during the operation, but it is the surgeon who sets the tone and the other team members who respond to it. The surgeon, after all, is responsible for the entire operation and his professional reputation is on the line every time he performs surgery.

The seven thoracic (chest) and cardiovascular surgeons on the staff of the Cleveland Clinic Foundation, widely considered among the world's best, have spent many years of training and gained much experience in their specialties. Their occupation may be considered glamorous, but a tremendous amount of hard work is involved. The average Foundation cardiovascular surgeon puts in five twelve-hour days a week, including many hours standing at and bending over operating tables, working with intense concentration. (Open heart surgery typically takes from three to six hours, and about seventy-five operations are performed every week at the Cleveland Clinic.) About 10 percent of the bypass operations performed here are "re-dos," or second operations, which are technically more difficult to perform. Also, many of the surgical patients are referred to the Cleveland Clinic by doctors at other hospitals because they are especially complex cases that require the utmost expertise.

The surgical fee for these operations at the Cleveland Clinic, which is generally on a par with other large hospitals, amounts to a lot of money, but if you believe you or your insurance company are personally enriching the surgeon with this fee, you are mistaken. Though Cleveland Clinic surgeons are paid very well, the Clinic is a group practice, which means that surgery fees, like other fees, go into the Foundation's combined revenue, rather than directly to the surgeon. It also means that a sizable portion of the surgery fee income is used to support the extensive research the Foundation conducts on heart disease and other medical problems.

The first stop for the surgeon is the scrub sink; then he is helped into a green surgical gown and rubber gloves. Like other members of the team, he wears a sterile cap and mask. Fresh from viewing the patient's angiogram, he knows exactly where he is going to operate. He requests reports from other members of the team on the patient's vital signs and general condition. He examines

8. Open Heart Surgery

the work done so far and inspects the saphenous vein segment that was taken from the leg.

He first cuts a segment of the left internal mammary artery (LIMA) from inside the chest wall. It is a slow process, cutting away the strip of fatty tissue surrounding the artery so that the strip, encasing the artery, is freed and the end of the artery can be swung down to the heart. The upper part of this patient's left anterior descending artery, which supplies blood to much of the heart, is totally obstructed. Grafting the end of the left internal mammary artery to a point on the blocked artery below the obstruction brings a new blood supply to the heart. Many surgeons prefer to graft the end of this artery to the most important blocked artery, because, as noted earlier, experience has shown that the left internal mammary artery remains open after surgery longer than saphenous vein segments, in most cases. While the ongoing process of atherosclerosis results in obstruction of many saphenous vein bypasses after six or seven years, the LIMA tends to remain open, on average, for a decade or longer.

The surgeon cauterizes the small capillaries surrounding the mammary artery as he completely frees the required segment from the chest wall. Next, he requests another instrument and slices through the pericardium to expose the heart. At this point, the heart is still beating. He reaches into the cavity and lifts the pinkish-red moving organ, coated with yellowish fat, examining it for the tiny network of coronary arteries that lie on its surface.

At this stage, the patient must be put "on bypass," so that the beating of the heart can be stopped, and it can be worked on. Preparing for the heart-lung machine to take over the functions the heart and lungs normally perform, the surgeon cuts a number of clear plastic tubes to their required lengths and then clamps them to the cotton sterile drapery, where they will be at hand. Now he begins the first exercise of the delicate suturing that heart surgeons can perform so dexterously, often with either hand. He sews a small circle of purse-string sutures on the aorta, carefully gathering the loose ends of the threads and passing them through the thin plastic tubes to separate them so they are not mixed up with the other suture threads that will soon be leading from the heart and resting on the drapery. He forms a similar pattern of "holding" sutures on the wall of the heart's right auricle. Next, he makes a small incision in the aorta, places one of the plastic heart-lung machine tubes into the hole, and draws the purse-string sutures tight. This secures the tube to the aorta, which makes it possible for the heart-lung machine to return oxygenated blood to the patient's circulatory system. After the surgeon secures a similar tube to the right auricle, venous blood will be carried from the patient to the heart-lung machine. Now the blood can be circulated between the machine and the patient continuously, the oxygen-depleted blood traveling through the machine and picking up oxygen (while releasing carbon dioxide) and then returning to the body.

After a countdown, the heart-lung machine is turned

8. Open Heart Surgery

on, and its rotors begin to turn at low speed. The surgeon asks that a precalculated amount of heparin, which prevents blood from clotting, be inserted into the bloodstream. In any operation, blood clots must be prevented because they can block blood flow and even damage organs. In open heart surgery, there is usually little loss of blood, since it is recirculated through the heart-lung machine.

The surgeon checks the patient's temperature and mean arterial pressure on the monitors, then orders the perfusionist to cool the blood with the heart-lung machine. It is necessary to cool the patient's body to below-normal temperatures to slow the metabolism and to decrease oxygen requirements.

It is time to stop the heartbeat. The surgeon clamps the aorta, which stops the flow of blood and, in effect, separates the heart from the rest of the cardiovascular system. With a needle, he injects a cardioplegic solution (*plegia*, paralysis) directly into the aorta, which stops the heart. It slows gradually, contracting in an erratic fashion, until it stops in the middle of a beat. Then the surgeon injects more cardioplegic solution into the arteries below the blockages. The heart turns pale as the blood flow ceases. The surgeon checks various areas of the organ with a temperature probe to be sure the cold solution is doing its job everywhere it is supposed to.

A look at the monitors now shows a zero heartbeat. The temperature has dropped to 25 degrees Centigrade, from a normal of close to 40 degrees. The surgeon asks the heart-lung perfusionist what the blood flow rate is and is told that it is three liters per minute. If he wants the rate adjusted, it can be done quickly through the machine.

The surgeon picks up the still heart and examines its fat-coated surface carefully. He must locate the blocked arteries in the midst of the layer of fat—a task that requires training and experience, because the tiny arteries are not readily apparent. He probes the fat with an instrument and locates the obstructed left anterior descending artery. When he has chosen the point on this artery where the left internal mammary artery is to be grafted, he makes a small incision the same shape as the end of the artery, which has been clamped to prevent blood flow. Now he fits the end of the artery to the opening and quickly puts in a series of tiny sutures around the connection. To see this micro-suturing, he uses the special magnifying lenses attached to the glasses he wears. He checks carefully to be sure the connection is tight but not too tight. The stitches cannot be too close together or too far apart, and they must be positioned correctly.

The surgeon requests a section of the saphenous leg vein, which is in a container filled with fluid. He takes his time, inspects the vein very carefully, and then trims one end of it into the shape of opening he will need to match up with the hole he has already cut in the right coronary artery. This artery, too, is obstructed fairly high up and he has selected a point below the obstruction for the graft. He holds the saphenous vein upside down, so its one-way valves, which help keep the blood

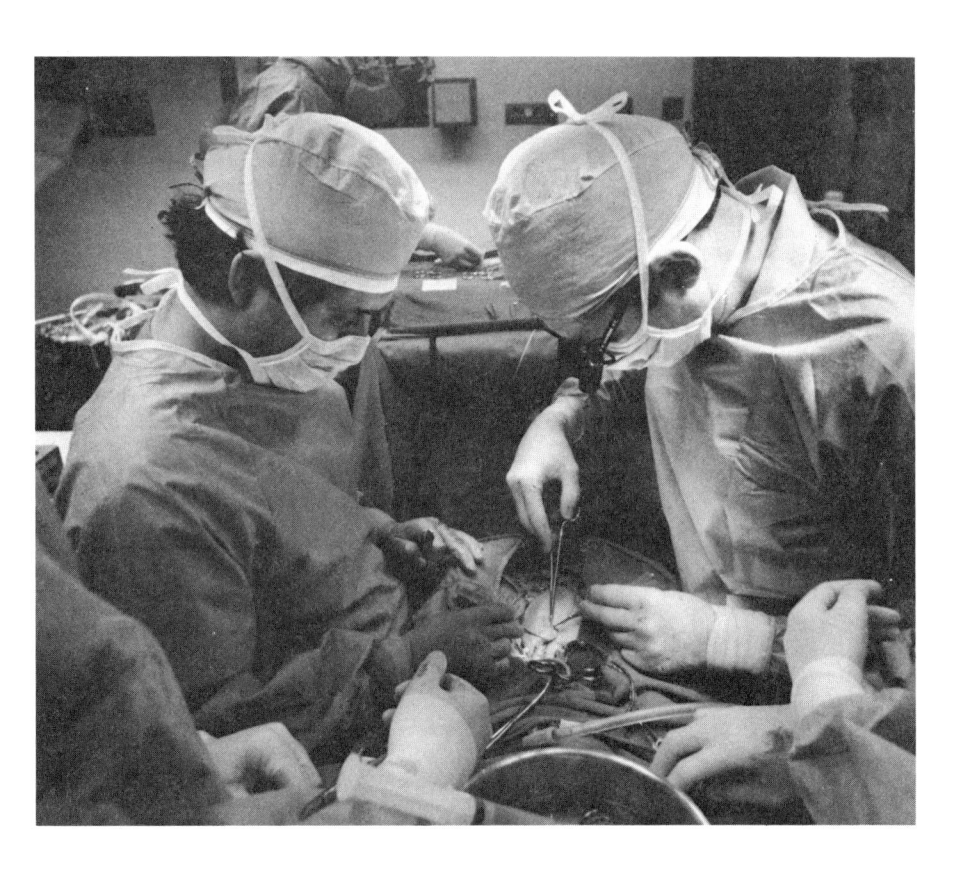

An open heart operation at the Cleveland Clinic. The surgeon, wearing special magnifying glasses, is the undisputed head of a team of ten or eleven skilled people, including one or two surgical resident physicians as well as cardiovascular nurse clinicians, scrub nurses, circulating nurses, anesthesiologist physicians and nurses, and a cardiovascular perfusionist to operate the heart-lung machine. The patient is draped from head to foot in sterile cloth; the only opening is the "surgical field," through which the heart operation is performed. The patient's head is beneath a draped frame supporting the holding pan in the foreground of the picture.

in the leg from flowing down, will not act as barriers to blood flowing to the heart. He cuts the vein to the desired length, then begins the delicate micro-suturing that will connect the lower end of the vein to the right coronary artery. He does not hold the small curved needle in his hand but rather grips it with a pair of long-handled forceps, sewing tiny stitches with the thin plastic thread. The deftness with which he handles the forceps and needle is awesome. This painstaking work takes him only a few minutes. Passing the stitches first through the vein and then through the artery incision, he draws the two tightly together, making about eight turns of the suture. Then he ties a series of tiny knots with one hand (some surgeons can tie these knots equally well with either hand) and pauses to inspect his work. He inserts a probe into the vein and slides it up and down, testing to be sure the vessel is fully open the way it is sewed on.

Now it is time to begin the third graft in this triple bypass operation. An assistant hands the surgeon another segment of the saphenous leg vein and he carefully inspects it and again cuts the end in a shape to match the incision he will make in the next obstructed artery. This one is the left circumflex artery, which carries blood laterally across the heart's surface to supply major areas not reached by the right coronary artery or the left anterior descending artery.

The surgeon repeats the suturing procedure after determining the optimum location for the graft in this artery. All the while, his surgical residents assist him,

8. Open Heart Surgery

keeping the dangling ends of sutures arranged in order on the drapery, holding tissue out of his way with instruments as he sutures in hard-to-reach places—acting as extra pairs of hands in a variety of ways. The other team members answer the surgeon's questions instantly as he checks on the patient's vital signs and general condition from time to time. "What's the blood flow?" "How much urine?" "Arterial pressure?" If a team member fails to respond instantly to the surgeon the quiet of the operating room may be broken with an angry reprimand. Anything even remotely resembling slackness is anathema to the surgeon, and it must be stamped out. The surgeon may crack a few jokes and chat amiably from time to time during the operation, but experienced operating room personnel know this is not an invitation to relax completely—and they do not.

"The people on our bypass surgery teams are the best in the business, from the surgical residents to the nurses and the technicians," says Dr. Paul Taylor with justifiable pride. A top cardiovascular surgeon who has performed more than 9,000 heart operations at the Cleveland Clinic, Dr. Taylor stresses that a surgeon can only achieve maximum effectiveness with a first-rate operating room team. "It's the team approach that counts in the final result," he declares.

The next step for the surgeon is to join the top ends of the two saphenous veins to the aorta. He places a metal clamp on this large vessel to separate a small area where the veins will be grafted. Then he punches two small openings and meticulously sutures the ends of the veins to the aorta. This will allow the oxygenated blood leaving the heart to travel from the aorta directly to the two coronary arteries, bypassing the obstructions in these vessels. Heart surgeons self-deprecatingly refer to their work as "fixing plumbing," and it is, if you disregard the marvelously sophisticated technology and surgical artistry involved. The final result of this complex surgery is arterial plumbing that works better.

After a final inspection of the grafts, the work of repairing the heart is finished. But this is not the time for the surgical team to relax, because the crucial step of bringing the patient off the heart-lung machine is next. The heart muscle, which has been cooled and temporarily paralyzed to keep it still, must be warmed up and made to take over the job of pumping the blood again. But the muscle is stiff and cold, and it takes a little time before it is ready. Sometimes the surgeon must take two electrical paddles, place them on the heart, and send a jolt of electricity into it to shock the muscle into action. When the operation has been long and complex, it can take several hours before the heart regains its full beating strength and the patient can be taken off the machine. In most cases, though, the electric shock works quickly. The heart begins beating in an irregular, spasmodic pattern, and the color of the muscle turns from pale pink to red.

The heart is still lying in the open cavity as it resumes beating, and the surgeon takes this opportunity to inspect the vein and artery grafts for any leaks as blood courses

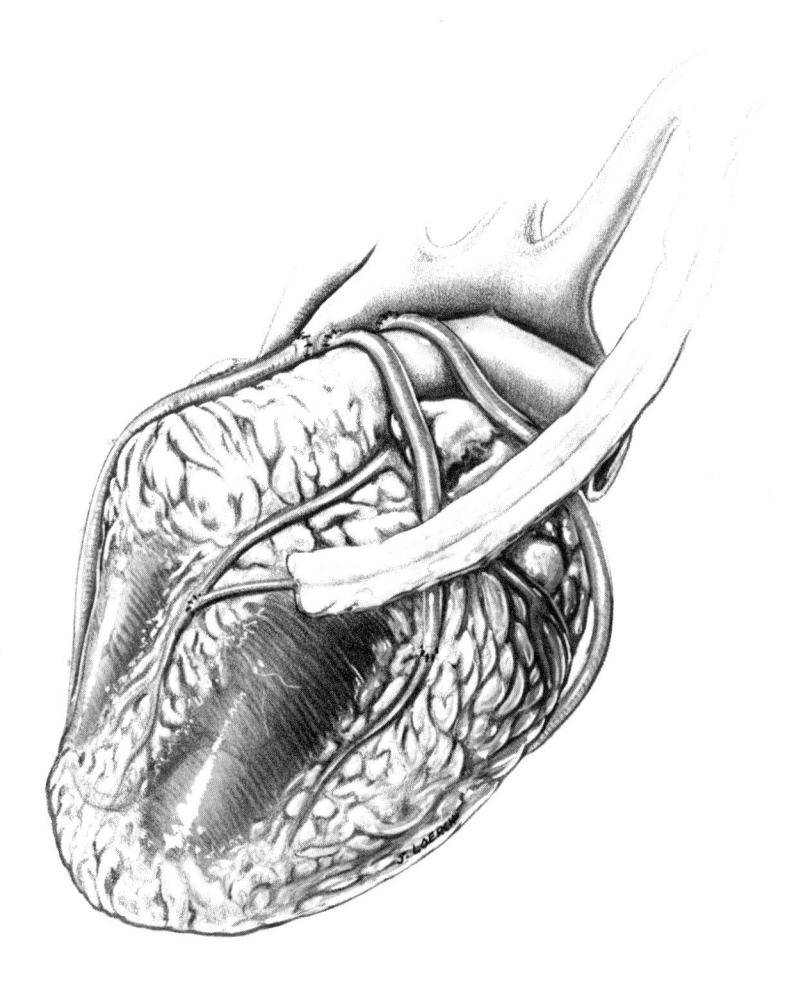

This illustration of a quadruple coronary bypass shows the end of an internal mammary artery (the large vessel coming from the right) grafted to the anterior descending coronary artery below the point at which it is blocked. In addition, three saphenous leg vein segments have been grafted to the aorta (*top*) to carry blood to points below blockages in the right coronary artery and the high lateral circumflex and the lateral circumflex coronary arteries.

through the vessels on the heart's surface. If anything were amiss, the operation would have to be halted and the patient put back on the heart-lung machine while repairs were made.

If everything is satisfactory, the surgeon and his assistants turn their attention to the monitors to observe the state of the patient's cardiovascular system. If the mean arterial pressure or the pressure inside one of the heart chambers appears to be too low, the surgeon orders more fluid to be delivered through the pump to correct the pressure. Sometimes a pacemaker is connected to the heart to increase the heart rate, which helps the heart perform better.

Now the efforts turn to stopping any further bleeding around the heart and the chest cavity before closing the cavity. With the amount of cutting that has been done, some tiny vessels are usually still oozing blood. The heparin the patient has been given, of course, facilitates bleeding, so at this point protamine, an antidote for heparin, is injected. Taking the electrical cautery in one hand, the surgeon examines the inside wall of the chest and the rest of the cavity, cauterizing each vessel that is still bleeding. The cavity must be dry before it is closed, though there will still be some bloody fluid released on the heart's surface and in the chest cavity after the incision is closed. Clear plastic tubes are inserted to drain off these fluids for a day or two in the recovery room. After satisfying himself that the bleeding has been stopped or controlled, the surgeon may order another

8. Open Heart Surgery

injection of protamine to help control any further bleeding.

At this point, the surgeon is finished with his work. He will leave the closing of incisions to the surgical residents and the rest of the operating room team. There is another patient in another operating room being prepared for him. This operation is just one of many that he performs, day in and day out. Yet it is no less important for that, and this is underscored by the way surgeons take their leave of the room. Most surgeons take a moment to congratulate the assistants on the team. "Good operation, doctor," they will say to each surgical resident, sometimes shaking hands with them over the operating table.

Now the surgical team completes the last stage of the operation, which is to close the incisions. The patient's heart is beating satisfactorily, the heart-lung machine has been disconnected, and the catheters have been removed. A surgical resident has sutured the left leg incisions with neat, subcutaneous stitches that will leave only four thin scars on the inside of the leg. The circulating nurse and the scrub nurse do a sponge count, the first of two. The surgical resident releases the U-shaped retractor, which permits the bringing together of the two sides of the patient's chest. With a rugged steel needle, the resident punches holes through the bone and inserts about a dozen stainless steel sutures, pulling them tightly to securely close the breastbone. The sutures will remain in place permanently, unless they are removed for a second open heart operation.

The resident closes the chest incision, usually with subcutaneous sutures that will not have to be removed because the material eventually disintegrates. The nurses have completed their two instrument and sponge counts before the incision is closed, and the operation is finished. The patient's body is slid carefully onto a rolling bed, which is pushed immediately to the recovery room, where nurses and technicians are waiting. The patient is connected to a breathing machine, even in the recovery room, because the body is still paralyzed and the patient is still unconscious from the anesthetic. Various catheters and monitors will continue to monitor some body functions. The patient may sleep deeply for six to eighteen hours after the surgery.

When the open heart operation is not coronary bypass surgery, it is most often the repair or replacement of heart valves. The preparations and procedures for opening and closing the chest are the same as those for bypass surgery, but valve surgery requires the surgeon to operate inside the heart, rather than on the surface vessels.

Most valve surgery is on the two valves on the heart's left side—the part of the heart that pumps oxygenated blood to the body. (See the earlier chapter "Nature's Marvelous Pump.") The mitral valve controls the flow of blood from the upper chamber (the atrium) into the lower left chamber (ventricle), which is the heart's main pumping chamber. The aortic valve controls blood flow from the left ventricle up into the aorta, the large "pipeline" through which the blood moves to the rest of the body. Any malfunction of these valves can cause serious

8. Open Heart Surgery

heart disease (see the earlier chapter, "Heart Disease: What Goes Wrong with the Pump").

Repair of a valve is preferable to replacement because it is simpler to do and the use of artificial tissue is not necessary. Sometimes a valve is not badly damaged, but its leaflets are too tight to permit normal blood flow. A surgeon can correct this malfunction without removing the valve from the heart, by spreading the tight leaflets apart with his finger or by cutting them apart. This frees up the too-tight valves. This procedure, called a commissurotomy, is most often done on the mitral valve. Sometimes the problem is a valve that leaks and allows blood to flow backward. To correct this, a surgeon stitches the leaflets partially together to narrow the opening. Another procedure is to suture a piece of material onto the leaflet to enlarge it, which makes it more effective in preventing the back flow of blood.

However, when a heart valve is severely damaged and beyond repair, it is usually necessary to replace it with an artificial valve. Medical science has developed artificial valves that, though they do not look like natural valves, perform their functions, allowing blood to flow through when open and stopping the flow of blood when closed. The three most common replacement valves are the disc valve, the ball-in-cage valve, and the tissue valve. The metal and cloth valve flips shut at an exact time in the heart cycle to prevent blood leakage while allowing blood to flow freely when open. The ball-in-cage valve, another simple-looking device, works like the ball valve that divers use on a snorkel tube. When the ball is raised, blood can flow through the valve. When the ball is dropped (in turn in the heart cycle) it prevents blood from flowing backward. The main problem with these mechanical valves is that blood clots can form in them. It is necessary for patients with mechanical valves to take anticoagulant medication (blood thinners) regularly for the rest of their lives.

Anticoagulants are not necessary, however, if a tissue valve is used as a replacement. This valve is sometimes called a porcine valve because the tissue is from the heart of a pig; it is chemically treated for use in human hearts. There are no exposed metal parts in it. The chief drawback to this valve is that it often tends to calcify, which causes the valve to deteriorate after about ten years. Patients with this type of valve have to consider the possibility that a second valve replacement operation will be required. Another potential problem is bacterial infection in the area of the new valve. Patients are given prophylactic antibiotics to prevent this.

Which type of valve is best for each patient depends on a variety of factors, including the fact that long-term anticoagulant therapy can be detrimental for some individuals, such as women who may wish to become pregnant. Usually several different types of valves are immediately available during an operation, and, after seeing the heart, the surgeon may choose a different valve from the one that was originally intended for use.

When a surgeon replaces an aortic valve, he makes an incision in the aorta near the valve. Working through this opening, he cuts the damaged or malfunctioning leaflets

8. Open Heart Surgery

of the valve and removes them, preserving only the firm ring that supported the natural valve. Then he inserts the replacement valve and stitches it in place. To replace a mitral valve, the surgeon must cut into the heart through the left atrium to reach the valve and then follow the same procedure, cutting away the leaflets and suturing the new valve securely in place.

In another open heart procedure, an aneurysm—a bulge in the wall of the heart, something like that which can appear in the weakened sidewall of an automobile tire—is removed. This weakening and bulging of the heart wall often occurs in the left ventricle, the heart's main pumping chamber. A large aneurysm can impair the pumping ability of the heart. To remove the aneurysm and improve the heart's pumping power, a surgeon cuts around the bulge and lifts out this stretched tissue. He then sutures the opening together. If the aneurysm is especially large, it may be necessary to sew on a patch of material, such as Dacron, which will remain permanently in place.

This same sew-and-patch procedure is used to repair septal defects—holes in the wall that separates the left and right sides of the heart. Some people are born with these defects, which permit blood to flow back and forth between the two sides and thus impair heart function. Cutting into the heart, the surgeon can reach this dividing wall and repair it by suturing the hole shut or by sewing on a patch, which eventually will be covered with new tissue and thus become a permanent part of the heart.

All these types of open heart surgery offer a better

quality of life and freedom from heart symptoms that plague many people. Only in the past two decades has this remarkable surgery been widely available to people everywhere, in hospitals all over the United States and in other countries. With heart disease so widespread, it is little wonder that this much-needed surgery has become one of the most common types of operations performed today.

9.
The Intensive Care Unit

At the Cleveland Clinic, it is called the Cardiovascular Intensive Care Unit. At other hospitals, it may be called the coronary care unit or the recovery room. Wherever it is, and whatever it is called, the place where patients first wake up after open heart surgery is specially designed and equipped to care for heart patients.

It is the place where patients first realize, gratefully, that they have survived their operations. But it is also a place where the patient feels pain, discomfort, helplessness, disorientation, and confusion, in part because of the effects of the anesthetic and medication and in part because of the strange environment.

You will be in a deep sleep for several hours following surgery because of the lingering effects of the anesthetic. Your breathing is still being done for you by a respirator, a machine that rhythmically pushes oxygen into your lungs through a breathing tube in your throat. This is necessary because the anesthetic relaxed your lungs and muscles and, until it wears off completely, the lungs can't do their job unassisted.

Your first conscious experience here is likely to be the sound of a nurse's voice calling your first name and telling you "Wake up—the operation is over." You may be in such a deep slumber that you don't want to wake up, but the voice is insistent. When you do rouse yourself enough to look around, you find yourself in a strange place that looks like a scene from a science fiction movie. At the Cleveland Clinic, and in many other large hospitals, you're in a room with maybe a dozen or more other patients, all of them connected up to a variety of wires and tubes. The room is crammed with all sorts of space-age machines, television monitors, buzzers, and beepers. The lights are always on, and it's hard to tell day from night.

You find that you can't talk because the breathing tube passes through your voice box. You have to rely on gestures to the nurses, or they may give you a pad and pencil if you want to write a note. You also have a nasogastric tube running through your nose to your stomach to drain stomach fluids. The catheter that was inserted into your bladder in the operating room is still there, connected to a container that measures your urine output (this shows how well your kidneys are working). As if these weren't enough, you discover that there are tubes protruding from your chest to drain the fluids that are leaking from the vessels that were cut during the operation. They are connected to bottles in a closed-drainage

9. The Intensive Care Unit

system that gurgles continuously. Then there are the plastic bags filled with fluids above you, each connected to the intravenous lines that were inserted in the operating room. These lines carry various medications directly into your bloodstream as needed. They also carry blood, if necessary, and glucose (a sugar solution), a form of nourishment.

If a pacemaker was used during your surgery, you may still have the wires in your chest, which may be connected to another pacemaker in the intensive care unit. And electrodes will be attached to your chest and connected to a electrocardiograph. The apparatus is connected to a monitor by your bed and to another monitor at the nurses's station. Your heart rate and heart rhythm will be monitored as long as you are in the unit. The system is equipped with an alarm that sounds if any unusual rhythm occurs and a device that starts printing the EKG as soon as the alarm sounds. The same alarm goes off if the heart rate decreases or increases too much. With this much monitoring and lifesaving equipment at hand, you could scarcely be in a better place if something goes wrong.

You soon find that you are being watched and checked in more ways than these, however. About every fifteen minutes, the nurse attending you takes your temperature, pulse, and blood pressure, checks your breathing pattern, and notes your skin color to see if it is returning to a healthier pink. The problem with all this attention is that it constantly disrupts your sleep, and you want to sleep more than anything else.

It is quite common for post-surgery patients to be disoriented in the intensive care unit. In this strange environment, you don't know whether it's night or day, and the lingering effect of the anesthetic sometimes includes confusion and loss of memory. The medication you are receiving also contributes to these conditions. Many patients don't remember much about the twenty-four or thirty-six hours they spend in the unit, even though they may remember nearly everything else about their hospital stay.

You ache all over, although the pain is not usually excruciating. What usually hurts most is coughing, and this is something the nurses will insist you do periodically after the breathing tube is removed, as you were instructed before the operation. It feels as though your chest will come apart (which, of course, it doesn't) and you are grateful for the nurse's suggestion that you hold a pillow to your chest while you cough. You are not as grateful, however, for the way she pounds your back while you cough, but this has to be done to loosen phlegm in the lungs so you won't get pneumonia.

The catheter in your bladder makes you feel as though the bladder is full. And you are very thirsty—after all, your mouth has been open for twenty-four hours or more —but you aren't allowed much to drink. The doctors don't want you to become waterlogged, and too much to drink can cause you to become sick and vomit, which would be very painful. Two sensations you don't feel are hunger and the need for a bowel movement, which is fortunate, considering your condition.

9. The Intensive Care Unit

If the pain becomes severe enough, you can request more medication from your nurse or one of the doctors who visit you periodically. Many types of pain-killing medication are available, and the medical personnel won't prescribe it in dosages that are addictive.

Patients can have complications in the intensive care unit, of course, depending on their condition. Medications, disturbances of body chemistry, and the trauma of surgery can affect the sinoatrial node, the nerve center in the heart that sparks the electrical impulse that makes the heart beat. This can also happen if the blood has too much or too little potassium or is too acidic. In some patients, this can cause the sinoatrial node to malfunction temporarily, which may make the heart beat too fast or too slow or erratically. Electronic pacemakers can correct these problems, as can medication. If the heartbeat should become too erratic and go into ventricular defibrillation, a dangerous condition, it can be shocked back to a regular beat with the same type of electrical paddles that are sometimes used to restart the heart in the operating room.

In a small number of cases, the heart may fail to work properly after surgery for other reasons. For example, if a newly grafted vessel closes and obstructs the blood flow, the left ventricle may not receive enough oxygen, and its pumping ability is impaired. This can lead to congestive heart failure, in which the blood backs up in the lungs because not enough blood is being pumped to the rest of the body. There are remedies readily available for such problems, including stimulants that make the heart beat more vigorously, blood vessel dilators to facilitate circulation, and diuretics to help the patient's body get rid of excess liquid. The heart can be made to beat faster and more forcefully by administering epinephrine, dopamine, or digitalis.

Another device is available in case these medications fail to correct the problem of a weakly pumping heart. The intraaortic balloon pump, a machine with a long, thin catheter, with a ten-inch-long balloon at the end, can help the heart pump blood until it is strong enough to pump adequately on its own. The end of the catheter is inserted into an artery at the groin and slid up into the aorta. Air is pumped by the machine into the balloon, which inflates, filling about 85 percent of the aorta's diameter. The action is timed so that the balloon inflates when the heart is in the resting phase. When this happens, the balloon forces the blood in the aorta into the coronary arteries and out toward other arteries, just as a healthy heart would pump it out. Then the balloon deflates when the heart contracts, which permits the blood to flow around it. The inflation and deflation of the balloon is regulated and synchronized with the patient's heart rate. The balloon pump may be used for several days, until the medication has acted to enable the heart to pump blood more effectively on its own. The catheter is then withdrawn, a painless procedure.

Cases of kidney failure, liver failure, and strokes have also been known to occur in intensive care units, but they are relatively rare and can be treated with medication

9. The Intensive Care Unit

and equipment at hand. Rarely, a heart attack occurs but usually can be treated with medication.

After the anesthetic has worn off completely and you are able to breath well on your own (usually within twenty-four hours), a nurse will remove the breathing tube from your throat. Now you can talk, although you may find your voice a little hoarse and your throat a little sore. The nasogastric tube is removed. To replace the breathing tube, you are given a small oxygen tube to wear, a lightweight device that hangs over your ears like a pair of glasses and has two short tubes that lead to the nostrils. Compared with the breathing tube, this device, which is connected to an oxygen supply, seems very comfortable.

At some point after you have been in the intensive care unit for a while, your spouse or other relatives are allowed to visit you. It is difficult to determine whether this visit will benefit either them or you, but it probably helps them because they can see with their own eyes that you are recuperating from the operation. You may be asleep when they visit, or you may not be fully alert and oriented as a result of medication. Some relatives are shocked to see their loved ones looking so terrible. The visit, however, can be a beneficial dose of love and affection for all concerned.

As you continue to recuperate, some of the other attachments to your body are removed. It doesn't hurt when the catheter is removed from your bladder, but you may have the sensation that your lower insides have been cleaned out with a vacuum cleaner. You may also have some burning or irritation for a short while afterward when you urinate. A nurse or doctor removes the drainage tubes from your chest with a quick yank, which doesn't usually cause much pain. Some of the intravenous lines are removed from your wrists. The tight bandages around the leg with the incisions are taken off, and the dressings on your chest incision are replaced with small patches. You are beginning to look and feel more like a normal human being again, and this helps your morale.

Coughing exercises continue, and breathing exercises begin, using the plastic ball-and-tube device you were given to practice with before the operation. Every two hours you are urged to inhale as deeply as you can through the plastic mouthpiece and see how long you can keep the ball up in the tube. Your lungs hurt, but you repeat this several times.

You are also encouraged to sit up in bed and to move your limbs around as often as possible; this includes swinging your legs over the side of the bed and letting them dangle. You will find that from here on, including the days you will spend in a regular hospital room after leaving the intensive care unit, the motto for patients is *Keep moving.* This is a vital part of your recovery, and it is one factor that you control. You won't feel like moving much at first, but it helps you if you force yourself to do it.

Years ago, physicians believed that prolonged bed rest was important for postsurgical patients, but experience has since shown that this is not true. In fact, the

9. The Intensive Care Unit

opposite is true: the sooner and more often a patient moves around after major surgery, the faster and better the recovery. If you are immobile, your body slows down, your breathing becomes shallow, and your lungs aren't active enough, and this can lead to pneumonia. Another hazard of immobility is that your circulation slows down, which can cause your blood to "pool" rather than move, and can cause blood clots to form in your leg veins. Blood clots can be dangerous, of course, because when they enter the circulation, they can obstruct the blood supply to your lungs, your brain, or your heart. In fact, immobility makes your entire body sluggish. Your intestines aren't active enough after you begin eating solid food again, and you become constipated. Your muscles are weakened as the result of prolonged bed rest, and it takes activity to restore them to their former capacity.

These are the reasons you should make activity and movement your goals when you leave the intensive care unit and transfer to a regular hospital room. *When* you leave the unit depends on your condition, but for many patients it is only one or two days after surgery. Now you are ready to take an active part in working for full recovery.

Before ending this chapter, one more subject should be discussed, because it might have an effect on the patient, as well as his or her relatives: temporary psychological disorders. The common experience of disorientation and confusion in the intensive care unit has been mentioned, but the psychological effects of surgery go further than that for some patients. It might not happen to you, but you—and especially your family—will be better prepared to cope with it if you know that it can happen and that it is temporary. These psychological effects can continue even after the patient leaves intensive care and returns to a regular room where he or she can receive visitors.

Danni Gogol Nadler, R.N., cardiovascular counselor at the Cleveland Clinic Foundation, explains: "These situations can cause a great deal of distress and concern for the family. One that people are least prepared for and find most disconcerting is when a patient is confused and disoriented. As a rule, most patients do very well with the postoperative experience because they have been briefed as to what to expect. Their recall of the first twenty-four hours or so after surgery isn't very good, but by that time they have regained some controls and leave the intensive care unit a short time later. Some patients seem to have more trouble than others: (1) those who may have disease in the vessels supplying the brain or other physiological process altering brain function; (2) those done as an emergency without any explanation about what is happening or briefing as to what to expect and no time to get used to the idea; (3) those who have a complicated course with a long intensive care stay; (4) those who normally are very assertive and aggressive in controlling their lives and others, are used to telling others what to do and having it done their way, and are competitive and time-oriented; and (5) those who have

9. The Intensive Care Unit

little or no symptoms and have not been ill with their disease.

"Patients who have 'post-op psychosis'—such as confusion, disorientation, belligerence, paranoia, hallucinations and the like—believe everything they think and feel. These beliefs usually center around conspiracies, torture, imprisonment or concentration camps, punishment, and sexual assaults or abuse. Whatever the case may be, patients see themselves as responding normally to an abnormal situation. Such patients may [and often do] say hurtful things to their family and act in an unbecoming manner. In fact, families often feel that the patient is not the same patient as before the surgery, and indeed, the patient is not. But the condition is temporary. Patients recover from this experience, usually without residual effects. They may never even remember any of it. Families remember everything; patients remember only what was true for them—which may have nothing to do with reality. An example is the patient who refuses to see or talk to anyone in his family and is angry at all the hospital staff—especially the nurses and doctors. He believes he is being tortured, while just outside the door his family is having a party. He feels his family is letting him suffer at the hands of these people while they are having a good time.

"I have learned that there is nothing that you can do to try to convince the patient otherwise. The patient truly believes that what he or she thinks is happening is reality. Though these delusions should not be reinforced, the patient needs to know that you accept the fact that he or she believes them. Even years later, when patients can say intellectually that they know that what they thought couldn't have been true, they nevertheless recall it that way. For them the events will never change. That was the way they experienced it, and that is OK; it doesn't have to change.

"The family usually needs a great deal of help with all of that. They need support to hang in there. The episodes are time-limited. Patients usually get better as they recover—as they get less medication and gain more control of their lives in a more normal life-style setting."

10.

Striving for Full Recovery

You are likely to feel elated when you are a postsurgical patient leaving the intensive care unit for the comfort of an ordinary hospital room. As an attendant pushes your wheelchair into the room, you consider this move to be proof that you have passed through the crucial early period of surviving your heart operation. From now on, the outlook is more optimistic—getting stronger every day and feeling less pain. The new room offers more comforts than intensive care, including television to watch and a more private atmosphere for visiting with your family.

When you first arrive, you are probably too weak to do anything more than stand up from the wheelchair and slide into the clean, comfortable bed. You sleep a lot during your first day or two here; it's more restful than intensive care, even though the nurses still wake you to check your temperature, pulse, and other things, as well as to give you medication.

You still have pain in your chest and the leg from which the saphenous vein was taken, and you may find that you wake up feverish in the night, with sweat-soaked pajamas. Fever is common after major surgery. Medication, including aspirin, is given to help control it. You will have a snug-fitting elastic stocking covering the lower part of the operated-on leg, and the ankle and foot on that leg will be swollen and sore. The surgical stocking helps to keep the blood in the veins from clotting and it is recommended that you continue to wear it after you get home from the hospital.

Besides the aches and pains, you will feel weak. You are soon encouraged to go to the bathroom by yourself, and some patients start taking showers the second day they are in the regular room, if they feel strong enough. If you are in an optimistic frame of mind, you are eager to begin doing such things for yourself. But you also find that each little activity wears you out completely and that you need to sleep immediately afterward. Still the knowledge that you can perform these little tasks is reassuring and leads you to want to try more.

You have no trouble getting the go-ahead to do this, as long as you are careful and pace yourself. In fact, the nurses are soon urging you to get out of bed and walk up and down the halls several times a day. The first time you attempt this a nurse may help support you, holding your arm as you totter gingerly along. You quickly run out of strength after a short distance and you are grateful for the comfortable bed you can slip back into. But the

10. Striving for Full Recovery

next time you try it you go a little further, and the distance keeps increasing in subsequent walks. With the nursing staff's encouragement, you may be walking two miles a day around the unit floor before you are discharged a week later.

Your plastic breathing toy has followed you to your room from intensive care, and you are urged to continue practicing deep inhaling with the device several times a day. You also continue to cough at intervals, with a nurse pounding you on your back to loosen the phlegm in your lungs.

You are now eating solid food—low-fat, low-salt, low-cholesterol meals. They are not very appetizing, especially since some of the medication you are taking tends to diminish your appetite and your sense of taste. But you need this nourishment, of course, to help you gain strength.

At the Cleveland Clinic, you are sent to a class with other recuperating heart patients to learn some of the do's and don'ts you must observe after you get home. Families of patients are encouraged to attend this class, since they will play important roles in helping the patient to recover fully and return to a normal life. You are making progress toward a full recovery, but your hospital stay after open heart surgery is usually only one week, and you will have to continue your recovery at home.

You are told that it is okay to shower and wash your chest incision (gently) and pat it dry with a towel. You are advised to keep wearing the surgical stocking for several weeks until the swelling in the leg goes down. It's a good idea to elevate your leg when sitting, and avoid crossing your legs, which interferes with circulation.

Airline travel is permissible, even when journeying home from the hospital, but you should get up every hour or so during the flight and walk for a few minutes. Riding in a car is fine, too, but again, if it is a long trip, the driver should stop every hour or so for a few minutes so you can walk around and stretch your legs. This activity keeps the blood circulation moving better and prevents the blood from pooling and clotting.

As for driving a car, your doctor will probably tell you when you can begin driving again, depending on your general condition. Most patients are told they may drive again after they have been home between three and six weeks. Driving is not a danger to your heart, but in a sudden stop or accident, your chest could hit the steering wheel, damaging the incision and possibly injuring your breastbone. This bone has been wired together, but it takes time for it to set, just as a broken leg does. You shouldn't chance interrupting this healing process.

Regular exercise is important to a good recovery, and this is stressed. You should continue daily walking after you get home, gradually increasing the distance beyond two miles if you feel comfortable doing it. In winter or rainy weather, it is suggested that you walk inside shopping malls, something that you see many heart patients doing in communities everywhere.

10. Striving for Full Recovery

Exercise also helps reduce emotional stress and promotes a positive attitude. Many, but not all, patients experience swings in mood and occasional days when they feel depressed after they return home. The causes of this experience aren't fully known. Some physicians believe it may be due to a temporary change in the body's chemistry following surgery; others attribute it to the patient's realization of what he or she has just gone through. Some people are fearful about being away from the expert medical care the hospital offers. But the feelings are temporary, and if they occur, they are part of the recovery experience.

To avoid or reduce depression and lethargy, doctors usually advise you to be as sensibly active as your energy permits. You should get up and out of bed every morning even though you aren't going anywhere. And you should get dressed, rather than stay in nightclothes all day. You should engage in such non-strenuous activities as hobbies, or visiting with friends or relatives. Take an interest in the news, what's going on in the world—anything but constant dwelling on your physical condition. If you have emotional concerns, it is good to talk them over with your family and close friends. A brisk walk is a good way to put emotional concerns in perspective and to feel better about yourself.

Though exercise is important, patients at the Cleveland Clinic classes are reminded that they should not attempt any activity that is too strenuous, such as lifting anything heavier than ten pounds for the first six weeks. And it is a good idea to avoid, permanently, exceptionally heavy lifting, such as that involved in shoveling heavy snow or picking up heavy furniture. In the first month after your operation, even such housework as vacuuming, bed-making, and gardening should be avoided. It is not likely to injure your heart, but stretching and bending might damage some sutures.

Some patients find that a supervised cardiac rehabilitation program helps them physically and psychologically, although it is not a requirement for most patients. Many hospitals and other medical centers offer such programs, and medical insurance often pays for them. An example is the outpatient cardiac rehabilitation program at St. Vincent Hospital in Toledo, Ohio. Patients are usually referred to the program by their physicians four to six weeks after their surgery. A stress test, blood test, and lean body mass weight analysis are performed to individualize the program for each patient. Then the patient returns three days each week for eight weeks for an hour of monitored exercise.

Each session begins with a physical assessment, then stretching exercises with weights, then work on stationary bicycles to increase arm and leg conditioning. Cool-down walking and stretching exercises complete the hour. The EKG and blood pressure are closely monitored throughout the sessions.

"Patients usually need the first two weeks to get adjusted to the program," says Ann Murawski, R.N., nurse coordinator. "After that we generally begin to see

10. Striving for Full Recovery

their endurance improve. We also encourage them to walk, ride bikes and maybe use predetermined weights on the days they don't come here to exercise."

At the end of the eight-week program, each patient is given an exercise plan to follow to continue his or her conditioning.

"We are trying to build these individuals physically through a monitored exercise program," says Ms. Murawski. "At the same time we are trying to build up their self-esteem. The patients are still dealing with the psychological factors of having heart surgery, and we have to educate them and give them a lot of encouragement. We deal with a lot of emotions. Our dietitians are involved, social workers help the family members, which is equally important, and support is provided by other departments of the hospital. We really make an effort to coordinate all of the needs of the patients in our program."

It is common for patients to be on medication for some time after open heart surgery. Your cardiologist or surgeon will decide what is required in your case, depending on your individual condition. He or she may prescribe one or more of a variety of medications that include nitrates, beta blockers, calcium channel blockers, diuretics, antiarrhythmics, antibiotics, antihypertensives, and anticholesterol drugs. Each is designed to treat a different symptom or condition. Some of these drugs produce side effects in some patients, but not in others.

You should ask your doctor about any medication

prescribed for you—what it is designed to do for you and what side effects it may have, if any. You should be scrupulous about following the directions of how often you should take it and how much you should take each time. And don't suddenly stop taking the medicine just because you feel better. That decision is best left to your doctor.

One of the most important topics on the minds of many postoperative patients is the resumption of sexual activity and the effects of surgery and its aftermath on that possibility. The medical facts are reassuring about resuming a normal sex life, but psychological factors do have a way of causing problems for a good many people, at least temporarily.

Physically, there are no particular hazards for newly repaired hearts in sexual intercourse. If you can walk two or three blocks briskly, which most postoperative patients can already do before they leave the hospital, you won't put any more strain on your heart during sexual intercourse. The usual physical changes that occur during sexual excitement and intercourse—faster breathing, increased heart rate, and higher blood pressure—are relatively mild and last only a brief time, just as they do in walking a couple of blocks at a brisk pace. Medical studies have proved this repeatedly.

A study of married couples conducted by Dr. Joseph G. Bohlen at the University of Minnesota School of Medicine showed that lovemaking in its various forms is really only light exercise. According to the study, noncoital sexual activity, such as stimulation of the genitals

10. Striving for Full Recovery

by the partner and self-stimulation, is the least stressful route to orgasm. In the three to six minutes before orgasm, the average pulse rate rose from 64 to 102—the equivalent of a slow walk. Coitus with the partner on top produced an average pulse rate peak of 110 at orgasm for the partner on the bottom. The average peak pulse rate for the partner on top was 127—less than that for brisk walking or mowing the lawn. And the peak pulse rate lasted only ten to sixteen seconds before going down. There were considerable variations for individual subjects, but the conclusion was that sexual activity carries a very small risk indeed.

About the only exception to this would be extramarital sex, which can be more stressful for several reasons. Guilt and fear of being found out add to emotional stress, as does the fact that extramarital sex often takes place in unfamiliar, rather than reassuring, surroundings. There is often an unexpressed need to perform well with a new partner, who may be younger and more vigorous. Sometimes there are the associated effects of too much food and alcohol intake, which add to the overall stress.

You may not feel strong enough to begin sexual activity when you first get home from the hospital, of course. The American Heart Association suggests that the majority of people who have had heart surgery are able to resume sexual relations one to three weeks after they are discharged from the hospital. The length of time will vary for each individual, of course, depending on that person's progress in recuperating.

Some medications, particularly those prescribed for

hypertension, can interfere with such sexual functions as erection and ejaculation. If you are taking such a medication and experiencing problems, you should tell your doctor about it. The doctor may change the medication to reduce or prevent these side effects.

Physical factors are not the cause of most sexual difficulties experienced by heart surgery patients, however. Psychological factors are much more likely to be the culprit. The two most common factors are fear about sexual performance and the general depression referred to earlier. With men, it is quite common and natural to feel reduced energy and desire in the early period after a serious operation like open heart surgery. The loss of physical strength is often accompanied by a fear of loss of virility, and this fear only makes it more difficult to perform. With women, there is the fear of being less sexually appealing because of surgical scars. Another fear is based on the unfounded myth that resuming sexual activity will often bring on a heart attack or cause death. If a patient isn't aware of all the medical evidence proving that this is false, he or she may worry needlessly. It is important to know that sexual relations after heart surgery are normal, desirable, and healthy. Lovemaking can produce a closeness, affection, and happiness that are of great benefit to the recuperating person, increasing his or her feeling of well-being.

The temporary depression felt by many postoperative patients produces unexplainable feelings of sadness and lethargy. Often the patient either has trouble sleeping

10. Striving for Full Recovery

or sleeps too much, especially during the day. Appetite may increase or decrease, as may body weight. Other common effects are chronic tiredness, lack of interest in life, and general irritability. According to the American Heart Association, this normal depression disappears within three months in 85 percent of cases. But while it lasts, it tends to exaggerate whatever previous sexual problems may have been present between husband and wife, and it certainly reduces the desire for lovemaking. This loss of desire, along with unwarranted fear that sexual activity may cause physical harm, may result in a couple needlessly stopping sexual relations for months or even years. If the depression continues beyond three months, a patient should seek counseling, which can help. Patients who remain depressed longer than this usual period after heart surgery have far less sexual activity and enjoy it less than those whose depression lifted earlier.

Good communication between partners can help prevent many sexual difficulties. A partner does not know what hurts or does not hurt the patient, and if not told, may be afraid to do anything. These things need to be talked about. A spouse may be overly protective of a heart patient, fearing to make any demands on the patient or not allowing him or her to be normally active. This attitude can reinforce the patient's feeling of being an invalid rather than a healthy recuperating person, which undermines his or her confidence. If you are the patient, you should realize that your illness and surgery has been an ordeal for your spouse, too. It is common for spouses to be anxious and depressed themselves, which can contribute to the overall tension in the marriage. Couples who discuss their sexual and emotional needs seem to have an easier time coping with any sexual problems that may arise.

There are some common-sense rules to follow when you first begin sexual activity after your heart operation. The first is choosing a time when you and your partner are rested and relaxed—maybe early in the morning after a good night's sleep or during the day after a nap. It is also best to wait one or two hours after eating a full meal. The process of digestion requires increased amounts of blood, which makes the heart work harder to pump even more blood required by your body for another activity. If you are taking nitrates (to dilate your coronary arteries) or other medication to help your heart function more efficiently, try to time your lovemaking so that you have taken the medication just before the sexual activity.

The American Heart Association suggests that a good way to resume sexual relations is with touching, holding, and caressing the other's body without the goal of orgasm, since this requires very little energy. A good many couples have found that these ways of expressing love and intimacy allow them to return slowly to a full sex life. As their self-confidence increases, they begin to feel more at ease with themselves and with each other without having to meet demands to perform. Don't try to

10. Striving for Full Recovery

push yourself to prove that "things are back to normal," advises the Association. Neither of you should expect too much at first; nearly everyone takes time to adjust to sexual activity after heart surgery. The best thing to do is approach sex slowly and just let this pleasurable part of your life happen.

You may be more aware than you ever were before of your increased heart rate, breathing, and muscle tension during sexual activity. But you should remember that these physical reactions are normal. If your chest or leg incision hurts in certain positions, try other, more passive positions to avoid pain and to conserve your strength. With a cooperative and understanding partner, sore incisions and muscles should not lessen the pleasure of lovemaking.

If you happen to be a patient whose heart does not yet have the ability to do its job sufficiently during sexual intercourse, you'll have symptoms that let you know it. Such symptoms include angina (the most common); pain in the jaw, neck, arm, chest or stomach; shortness of breath; and excessively rapid or irregular heartbeats. If you experience these, do not panic. Tell your partner, reduce your activity, rest, and take any medicine your doctor may have prescribed. When the symptoms go away, you can resume sexual activity. If they don't go away, you should call your doctor. A physician may decide that a small adjustment or change is needed in your medication or daily routine to help prevent these symptoms.

If physical factors are not limiting your sex life, but you and your spouse are having sexual difficulties, you should look at the emotional problems that can affect your relationship. A good sexual relationship, after all, also depends on other facets of a marital relationship. It is not uncommon for emotional stress to affect couples after one person has had heart surgery. If, for example, there has been a change in marital roles because the heart patient has had to give up a physically demanding job, insecurities can show up in both spouses. Family, legal, or financial problems can adversely affect a sexual relationship.

If any of these problems are affecting your sexual relationship, don't give up. Seek counseling with your spouse—it can help, as it has helped thousands of others. Ask your doctor to refer you to a qualified counselor; you have little to lose and a lot of happiness to gain.

By the time you have been home from the hospital for a month, you will probably feel much stronger and more energetic. Your muscles, which had gotten "out of practice" during your hospital stay and grown weak, will have regained a lot of their vigor if you have been exercising daily. If you had angina before your surgery, you probably are free of it now, or at least you don't have it as often and as severely as you did before. The aches in your chest and leg incisions have largely disappeared and you are feeling less like an invalid and more like a normal person. About this time, you begin looking forward to the day when you can return to work, if you have a job. The better you feel, the more you begin to

10. Striving for Full Recovery

relish the challenges of the active life you led before your surgery.

However, you still have to wait until your surgeon or cardiologist can check on the results of your surgery and the progress you have made in recuperating. At the Cleveland Clinic and many other hospitals, postoperative patients are usually advised to have a thorough checkup about six weeks after their surgery. If you live within reasonable traveling distance of the hospital, you can return there to be examined by your surgeon or cardiologist. If not, a cardiologist in your home community can perform the examination if the medical reports of your surgery have been forwarded to him.

The checkup will include laboratory tests and a thorough examination. Besides the standard resting EKG, you will take an exercise stress test and possibly other diagnostic procedures such as a thallium stress test. The checkup will probably require most of a day, including interviews with one or more doctors and nurses who will ask questions about any symptoms you have had, the side effects of any medications you have been taking, the amount of exercise, and so on.

On the basis of your postoperative history and examination and test results, your surgeon or cardiologist will tell you when it appears that you can return to work. One factor influencing the decision will be the type of job you are returning to. If it is a desk job, you will probably be able to return to work sooner than if your work involves physical exertion. If your job includes really heavy physical labor, you might be better off looking for a less physically taxing job. The same might be true if you have a desk job that involves a great deal of rush activity, tension, and emotional stress. Although some people seem to thrive on stressful jobs, you might be the type of person who is negatively affected by stress.

If there is any doubt in your mind, you should talk about it with your doctor, whose training and experience can provide valuable insight into the situation. In fact, the advice of your doctor, who is dealing with your individual condition and situation, should take precedence over any of the general guidelines for recovery described in this chapter. They are not intended to be definitive for any patient. Your doctor is the professional who can best help you to return to a full, active, and satisfying life.

11.
Adopting a New, Healthier Life-Style

WHEN YOU HAVE fully recuperated from open heart surgery, you will probably feel as though you have a new lease on life. You are likely to feel better than you have in years—more energy, fewer or no symptoms, and a more positive outlook. It is very likely that you will feel grateful for the impressive skills and knowledge of the surgeons and cardiologists who perform this miracle surgery to improve the lives of people with heart disease. At the same time, though, you should keep in mind the sobering fact that you still have heart disease, which continues to progress. Medical skills have brought you to the symptom-free state where you are now, but they can't keep you in this state indefinitely. The rate at which your underlying heart disease progresses may be very slow or very fast; there is no accurate way to predict this. But there is sufficient medical evidence to suggest that reducing your risk factors may help to delay the progression of the disease and forestall the appearance of symptoms. The surgeon and the cardiologist have done their jobs; reducing your risk factors and prolonging your improved physical state is *your* job.

You can't do anything about such unmodifiable risk factors as age, sex, or family history of heart disease. But hypertension, diabetes, and high blood levels of cholesterol and triglycerides can be modified with medication and diet. And with willpower and a positive attitude, you can change such factors as smoking, inactivity, obesity, and emotional stress.

To remind yourself of what these risk factors do to contribute to heart disease, you should pause here and go back and read the chapter "Look at Your Risk Factors." Even though medical science has not yet established final, conclusive proof of the effects of some factors, the weight of the evidence gathered thus far is reason enough to conclude that it would be prudent to eliminate or reduce those risk factors in an effort to forestall the recurrence of heart disease problems. Changing these factors can't hurt you and can bring you the additional benefits of feeling fit, looking better, and having a more positive attitude about yourself.

CIGARETTE SMOKING

This is one risk factor that nearly all physicians agree contributes significantly to heart disease. Since the death rate from heart attacks is 50 to 200 percent greater in heavy cigarette smokers than in nonsmokers, it is obvious that smoking is one of the key risk factors to be

11. Adopting a New, Healthier Life-Style

eliminated. If you do give it up, the risk will gradually decline to the same level as that of nonsmokers. Giving up smoking can be difficult. It is easier to quit, of course, when a doctor informs you that you have lung cancer or emphysema and your health has been ruined. With heart disease, you may be ruining your health by smoking, too, and it's best not to wait until it's too late before quitting. The fact that you have heart disease should be enough reason to launch you into an all-out effort to quit smoking. Call on whatever help you can get. The American Heart Association has a free booklet, *How to Stop Smoking*, which includes a five-step program. (Write to the American Heart Association, 7320 Greenville Avenue, Dallas, Texas 75231.) Join a Smokenders program, sponsored by the American Cancer Society, which uses behavior modification and facts to help people gradually quit the habit. Call your local chapter of the American Cancer Society for information.

HYPERTENSION

This important risk factor can be controlled, but your doctor can't do it alone; it takes your active participation to be successful. Hypertension interacts with other risk factors, such as smoking, obesity, lack of exercise, and emotional stress, and these factors can adversely affect your blood pressure. Statistics show that many people who have high blood pressure are also overweight. If you are overweight, you should follow a diet to reduce your caloric intake, and you should also exercise daily.

When you lose weight, your blood pressure often goes down simultaneously. In addition, exercise can help reduce blood pressure and also help to relieve emotional stress, another contributor to hypertension. You should, of course, try to avoid emotional situations that may cause your blood pressure to rise. Too much alcohol can also increase your blood pressure.

If you have hypertension, your doctor may advise you to restrict the sodium in your diet. Though many foods contain sodium, reducing salt intake is the most effective way to reduce your sodium consumption. Canned, frozen, and precooked foods contain large amounts of sodium, as do such luncheon meats as bologna and salami and such smoked meats as ham, sausage, bacon, and corned beef. Condiments like catsup, barbeque sauce, chili sauce, and mustard are loaded with sodium, too. The best way to cut your sodium intake is to avoid these foods, throw away your salt shaker, read the labels on canned foods, and switch to buying and cooking fresh foods. It will not be easy to give up some of your favorite foods, but there is a lot of room for tasty foods in a salt-restricted diet. A number of good cookbooks that concentrate on salt-restricted diets are available.

You can keep yourself healthier and possibly prolong your life by following these guidelines offered by the American Heart Association: (1) Keep appointments regularly with your doctor to see how your body is being affected by your hypertension and what kind of treatment plan is best for you. If your doctor prescribes medi-

11. Adopting a New, Healthier Life-Style

cations, take them exactly as instructed and keep taking them as long as the doctor says you should. Take care not to run out of pills, even for a single day. (2) Tell your doctor exactly how you are feeling, so your medication or diet may be changed if necessary to improve your condition. (3) Follow your doctor's advice about rest and relaxation. You will be advised on how much rest and relaxation you need and the kind of exercise you should or should not do.

OBESITY

The typical American diet and the lack of exercise result in a great many Americans being overweight, so trying to lose weight is probably the most common effort to improve health these days. You can look around you and see all manner of organizations and programs devoted to helping people lose weight; you have a wide selection to choose from. The one thing you shouldn't do, however, is resort to "fad" diets, which are ineffective in the long run and may even harm you. Weight Watchers is a respected organization that offers programs that have worked for many people. Exercise, when combined with a reduced-calorie diet, can help you lose weight; and there are many health clubs and exercise programs you can join.

The most intelligent thing to do, however, is to ask your doctor for guidance in losing weight before undertaking any diet or exercise program. The doctor may recommend a specific weight-loss diet and/or exercise program that is best for you. Watching your weight is an important part of a new, healthier life-style, since obesity is one of the risk factors that you can control. It may require a change in your daily eating habits, but this can be accomplished over a period of time with determination and the cooperation of your spouse and family.

The American Heart Association offers some useful tips to make it easier for you to reduce your calorie intake: (1) Keep a record of what you eat and when you eat it. Check it against your dietary plan and note any particular changes. Record the calories as you eat. An inexpensive calorie counter or calorie chart is available in any bookstore and in most supermarkets. (2) When shopping for food, *always* shop from a list and do the shopping *after* you have eaten. Do not buy foods that are likely to be a problem for "snacking" or are particularly tempting and are high in calories. (3) Try to eat three meals a day, at fairly regular times. (4) Eat in only one place in the house and don't do anything else while you are eating. (People sometimes forget they have eaten if they are absorbed in something else at the same time.) (5) Make portion sizes smaller and make them look more appealing by serving them in smaller-than-usual dishes and bowls. (6) Make second helpings hard to get by keeping extra food off the table and in the kitchen. (7) Eat slowly and chew your food well. Lay your fork or spoon down between bites. Try to be the last person eating at the table. Allow at least twenty minutes to eat

11. Adopting a New, Healthier Life-Style

and enjoy a meal. (8) Keep a variety of low-calorie foods on hand. These can include celery sticks, radishes, carrots, low-calorie gelatin desserts, and fresh fruit. If you like midday or evening snacks, plan to save something from each meal for a snack. (9) When eating out, choose roasted or broiled foods and ask that sauces and dressings be eliminated or served on the side.

CHOLESTEROL

This, of course, is the coronary risk factor that virtually all heart patients hear about and are warned against. Though your body manufactures a substantial amount of the cholesterol in your blood, there is good medical evidence that the level of cholesterol in the blood can be reduced by restricting the dietary intake of this substance.

How can you go about reducing your intake of cholesterol? Again, the best source of advice may be your doctor. At the Cleveland Clinic and other medical centers, nutritionists can provide complete low-cholesterol dietary plans and information on the cholesterol and fat content of various foods. Detailed printed information is available free from the American Heart Association. A number of nutrition books for heart patients are sold in bookstores; one of the best is the *American Heart Association Cookbook*, published by David McKay Company, New York.

The detailed printed information mentioned above can greatly increase your general knowledge of cholesterol. Most people have heard, for example, that eggs are one of the most concentrated sources of cholesterol. An average egg contains about 250 milligrams of cholesterol, all of it in the yolk. Since the American Heart Association recommends limiting cholesterol intake to 300 miligrams a day, whole eggs wouldn't be a good food choice. A three-ounce serving of red meat contains about 100 milligrams of cholesterol. The meats most heavily laden with cholesterol are the organ or variety meats such as brain (2,675 mg per three ounces), kidney (375 mg), and liver (300 mg). You can do much better by eating chicken and turkey, which have only 65 mg per three-ounce serving. Grains, fruits, and vegetables have no cholesterol; it comes only from animal sources.

The different types of fats in foods affect the way the body processes cholesterol. Saturated fat, the type that is usually solid at room temperature, can be harmful because it stimulates the production of low density lipoproteins, the "bad" fraction of cholesterol associated with a higher risk of heart disease. High levels of saturated fat are present in red meat, animal fat, such whole milk and dairy products as cheese and butter, hydrogenated shortenings, coconut and palm oils, and baked goods, snack foods, and non-dairy creamers made with coconut and palm oils.

Polyunsaturated fats, which are liquid at room temperature, can be beneficial in limited amounts. They can lower the total cholesterol level, and it is a good idea to substitute these for saturated fats when possible. Corn, soy, safflower, and other vegetable oils are examples of

11. Adopting a New, Healthier Life-Style

polyunsaturated fats. Many margarines contain these fats.

A third type of fat, called monounsaturated, is believed to be even more beneficial than polyunsaturated, which lowers both low density lipoproteins and high density lipoproteins, the "good" cholesterol fraction associated with lower risk of heart disease. Monounsaturated fat, found in olive oil, corn oil, and some kinds of safflower oil, appears to lower the "bad" low density lipoproteins but not the "good" high density lipoproteins in the blood. So a certain amount of olive oil may be good for you.

Still, it is believed that the total amount of all kinds of fat in the diet should be limited. Some 40 percent of the average American diet consists of fat. Based on study results, the American Heart Association recommends that the total amount of fat in the diet be reduced to 30 percent, with no more than one-tenth of the fat saturated fat. Other nutrition experts have urged even lower percentages of fat, especially saturated fat. The late Nathan Pritikin, founder of the Pritikin diet and the Pritikin Longevity Centers, believed in limiting total fats to 10 percent of the diet. He achieved impressive results in the people who stayed four weeks at his Longevity Centers; they lowered their average serum cholesterol from 235 to 175 in that short time. The Pritikin diet allows a little meat, fish, and poultry, but emphasizes complex carbohydrates—vegetables, fruit, and grains. Most physicians would concede that the Pritikin diet is very effective in lowering cholesterol levels, but many doctors believe that most Americans would find the diet too extreme to follow for long periods of time. If you can do it, though, the diet could be very beneficial.

Since red meat contains not only high amounts of cholesterol but also saturated fat, many medical experts recommend that heart patients reduce their consumption of it. Recent study results, however, have indicated that seafood, including shrimp, lobster, and salmon, which have a fairly high cholesterol content, actually helps prevent heart disease. The reason is that seafood has been found to contain a type of polyunsaturated fat that is different from that found in vegetables. This special fat can drastically lower serum cholesterol and fat levels. One study showed that people who eat an average of one ounce of fish daily were less than one-half as likely to die of heart disease as those who never eat fish. It is also known that Greenland Eskimos, who consume about fourteen ounces of fish every day, including seal fat and whale blubber, have a remarkably low incidence of heart disease. Researchers do not yet fully understand the biochemical reasons for this effect, but studies are continuing. In the meantime, it appears that eating seafood frequently may help prevent heart disease.

Several medical studies have suggested that a moderate consumption of alcohol—two or three drinks a day—raises high density lipoprotein levels associated with lower risk of heart disease, while lowering harmful low density lipoproteins. There is some evidence that moderate social drinkers have a lower incidence of heart

11. Adopting a New, Healthier Life-Style

disease than either teetotalers or heavy drinkers. Fiber, particularly oat cereal, has been shown in some studies to reduce the levels of low density lipoproteins. Other cereal grains may have the same effect. In fact, the American Heart Association recommends that while Americans are reducing the amounts of fats in their diet, they should increase the amounts of complex carbohydrates, which include cereals, whole-grain bread and pastas, beans, fresh vegetables, and fresh fruit.

Another type of blood fat believed to be harmful at high levels is the triglycerides. (See the earlier chapter "Look at Your Risk Factors.") Unfortunately for those heart patients with a sweet tooth, sugar raises the level of these triglycerides. Alcohol also raises triglyceride levels, while exercise lowers them.

One other substance, commonly ingested by most people, has been shown to help protect against heart attacks. That is plain old aspirin, a staple in most homes for many years. Several studies have indicated that aspirin can be effective in preventing the formation of clots in arteries, which are responsible for heart attacks. As little as one tablet a day seems to be effective.

EXERCISE

The role of exercise and its beneficial effects for heart patients were discussed at length in the earlier chapter on risk factors. You definitely *should* include exercise in your daily routine as part of a healthier life-style. In addition to its possibly direct benefit in slowing the progression of heart disease, exercise can help to reduce several other coronary risk factors. It is important in reducing and controlling your weight and your blood pressure. It also helps to relieve emotional stress, another risk factor, and, by making you more physically fit, it can improve your self-image and your outlook on the world. Exercise is also known to raise the levels of the beneficial high density lipoprotein fraction of your serum cholesterol. And it has been shown to reduce the level of triglycerides in the blood.

Too much exercise, or the wrong kind of exercise, can be harmful, of course. You should talk to your doctor before undertaking any kind of exercise program, since he or she is familiar with your condition. Many physicians recommend brisk walking as the best type of exercise for their heart patients. Jogging may not be ruled out if your condition allows it, and your doctor will set limits for you. Swimming, bicycling, and tennis are often recommended for people with heart disease if they will be pursued in moderation.

The most beneficial type of exercise, from a cardiovascular view, is one that is rhythmic, repetitive, involves the use of large muscles, and challenges the circulatory system. Only those exercises that significantly increase the blood flow to the working muscles for an extended period of time promote cardiovascular fitness—a state of body function that allows a person to exercise vigorously for long periods without undue fatigue and to respond to sudden physical or emotional demands more

11. Adopting a New, Healthier Life-Style

readily and with less strain. This is the goal of such exercise.

However, you should start slowly and gradually increase your level of exercise over a period of time, perhaps several weeks. You should choose the kind of exercise you will enjoy, or at least find rewarding, so you will want to continue. It should be demanding but not exhausting. You may want to do a kind of exercise that you can pursue conveniently on your own, or you might choose to enroll in a supervised exercise program. If you lose interest in one kind of exercise, switch to another kind, but by all means continue to get some form on a daily or a near-daily basis. It is important to your general health.

Many postoperative heart patients begin a daily exercise routine enthusiastically, but as the months go by, they encounter two obstacles: fitting the exercise conveniently into their daily routine and boredom. If you have a full-time job and you are busy with social and family activities in your spare time, you may indeed find it inconvenient to find a good time in your day for exercise. And if the exercise you've chosen requires you to get out of the house and go somewhere to do it, you may soon find yourself making excuses about why you can't do it today. Before long, you are skipping more and more exercise sessions, and you lose the fitness you have already achieved.

The American Heart Association points out that exercise must be a lifetime commitment, because when it is stopped, the beneficial effects on your cardiovascular system are rapidly lost. In effect, all your previous hard work and conditioning is wasted if you stop. To succeed in the long run, you must make exercise a *habit* with a definite place in your life.

There are ways to do this, of course. Since we are all creatures of habit in our daily routines, with a little determination you can *make* a place in your day for the habit of exercise. If inconvenient locations and bad weather are obstacles to your chosen exercise, you might rethink your plan and consider this alternative: Buy a motorized treadmill for walking and jogging, to place in your home. This has solved the problem of inconvenient locations and bad weather for a good many postoperative heart patients, including the author of this book. With this machine, it is easier to fit an exercise habit into your daily life—you don't have to leave the house, so the time required is shorter; bad weather doesn't interfere; and best of all, you don't have to be bored. Stationing a portable television set in front of the machine makes it possible to watch the news or become absorbed in a favorite program while you walk or jog. The time goes by so quickly that you hardly notice, whether your scheduled exercise time is thirty, forty-five, or sixty minutes a day.

The motorized treadmill, about six feet long with a moving belt to tread on, has certain advantages over the less-expensive, non-motorized treadmills you see advertised in magazines. You can set an exact speed on it, from

11. Adopting a New, Healthier Life-Style

slow walking to ten miles an hour jogging, and the speed remains constant while you exercise unless you want to change it. This helps you to set standards and gives you an accurate measurement of your performance. This isn't possible with the cheaper, non-motorized versions. You move the belt yourself on these, and some owners have complained that the rollers under the belts on some of these machines are uncomfortable.

A motorized treadmill is a considerable investment, since it generally costs about $2,000, but that is how you should look at it—as an investment in your long-term health that is well worth it. You probably wouldn't hesitate to pay several times this price for an automobile or for home improvements, and you should look at the purchase of a motorized treadmill—and its importance—in relation to such expenses.

If you enjoy bicycling as an exercise, you can accomplish the same thing at much less expense by purchasing a stationary exercise bicycle and placing a television set in front of it. But it depends on your own exercise preferences. Many people find they don't enjoy bicycling when they can't do it outdoors and enjoy the scenery on their ride. There are thousands of unused stationary bikes in homes everywhere, whose owners stopped using them after a few months.

Motorized treadmills and exercise bicycles are often advertised in sports, fitness, and runners' magazines. Many sports and bicycle shops have literature on them and can order one for you.

EMOTIONAL STRESS AND "TYPE A" BEHAVIOR

As mentioned earlier, heart specialists have long recognized emotional stress, and an individual's reactions to it, as a risk factor in heart disease. This risk factor is important enough for you, as a recuperated heart surgery patient, to take whatever steps you can to reduce it. It might mean changing jobs, for example, if your present position involves such stress that it is potentially harmful. Family relationships might have to be worked out so that emotional stress is reduced. You should examine the environment in which you live and work and look for ways to reduce stress if there is sufficient stress to damage your health in the long run.

And you should also take as objective a look as possible at yourself and the ways you react to stress. You may be able to change the potentially harmful ways in which you react in stressful situations. For example, if you are a "type A" personality, impatient, always trying to do too many things at once, striving for material goals or status, you might reassess your priorities. Many hard-striving, impatient people find it easier to do this after they realize that they have heart disease. Facing their own mortality for the first time in their lives, they begin to think in terms of the limited years they may have left to live. Often they conclude that some of their former goals and attitudes are not as important anymore, and other goals, such as relaxation and enjoyment of life with their families, are more important. Many such people find a serenity and happiness they had not known before, and they live fuller lives.

11. Adopting a New, Healthier Life-Style

Professional counseling can help you to achieve this change and reduce the risk factor of emotional stress. If you feel you need help, ask your doctor to recommend a counselor. It is an investment that could pay handsome dividends as an important part of your new, healthier life-style.

12.
What's Ahead in Treating Heart Disease

THERE HAS BEEN an incredible increase in the understanding and treatment of heart disease in the past few decades, and it is continuing. Medical research is being pursued by large numbers of professionals at centers all over the world, and the advancements resulting from their efforts will continue to improve the diagnosis and treatment of this most prevalent disease in the industrialized world. Already such advances as improved diagnostic equipment and techniques, new medications, and better emergency care have contributed to a 25 percent drop in the death rate from heart disease in the United States over the past decade. Open heart surgery has also played a role.

Many medical professionals believe that the public's greater knowledge of the causes of heart disease has helped, too. Smoking and the consumption of high-cholesterol, high-fat foods have declined somewhat, and

12. What's Ahead in Treating Heart Disease

more people are interested in exercise and fitness. There is still much progress to be made in altering the average American diet, which continues to be too high in saturated fat and cholesterol, and there are still too many people who are overweight and sedentary. But these coronary risk factors are being reduced by increasing numbers of people, a hopeful sign for the future.

In the area of diagnosis, advanced equipment and techniques are being perfected and put to use in new facilities for patients. At the Cleveland Clinic Foundation, for example, four new cardiac laboratories, built at a cost of one million dollars apiece, are being used not only for cardiac catheterization and arteriography but also for the application of a new, computer-based diagnostic technique, digital subtraction angiography. In this noninvasive technique, a small amount of dye is injected into a vein. The dye travels through the bloodstream and is "scanned" by computerized equipment at a selected area of the circulatory system. The computer then subtracts the radiographic frames containing images of bone from subsequent X-rays so that only the image of the blood vessels remains. Exceptionally clear images result, which make it possible to locate obstructions in such vessels as the carotid arteries, which cause strokes. Digital subtraction angiography cannot yet be considered a substitute for coronary angiography performed with a catheter because the images it provides do not produce adequate contrast visualization of the coronary arteries. Thus, it is not possible to visualize the exact anatomy of the coronary arteries as catheterization does. But the potential for further development and application of this new technique is very promising as another resource in the diagnosis of coronary disease. It has proven to be an excellent diagnostic tool for the evaluation of heart defects.

At the new Cleveland Clinic cardiac laboratories, patients who have abnormalities in their hearts' electrical conduction systems will have the benefit of sophisticated diagnosis aided by advanced physiological recorders and electrophysiological stimulators.

The laboratories are also equipped to allow doctors to stop some heart attacks in progress by injecting new clot-dissolving drugs through a catheter directly into the blocked coronary arteries. Streptokinase, urokinase, and a substance normally produced by the body, tissue plasminogen activator (TPA), are three of the clot-dissolving substances in various stages of testing and use in a number of medical centers. If such clot-dissolving drugs could be administered soon after heart attacks begin, many lives might be saved.

Research continues on new nonsurgical techniques for improving the blood flow in obstructed coronary arteries. One technique in use at the Cleveland Clinic and other medical centers is called balloon angioplasty. Angioplasty is an extension of the cardiac catheterization procedure. The word *angioplasty* means the remodeling of a blood vessel. When performed in the heart, it is known as percutaneous transluminal coronary angioplasty or

12. What's Ahead in Treating Heart Disease

the remodeling of a blood vessel in the heart, from the inside of the vessel, using a catheter inserted through a small puncture in the skin.

To perform angioplasty, the cardiologist uses a small catheter with an inflatable balloon packed tightly in the tip. The catheter is fed through the larger catheter used in the cardiac catheterization procedure until it reaches the narrowed areas of a coronary artery. The tip is then inflated by a hand compressor attached to the catheter. The inflated balloon presses the atherosclerotic plaque against the artery wall, flattening it and opening the vessel so that blood may flow through it more freely.

The premise is simple, but the procedure is not easy to perform. Since angioplasty is a relatively new technique, the number of cardiologists trained in the technique is still small. Manipulating the catheter through a tortuous maze of blood vessels takes skill and patience. The cardiologist cannot see these arteries on the monitor screen except for the few seconds after a dye is injected to show the obstructions. Once the doctor positions the balloon within the narrowed area of the artery, he must decide how much pressure will expand the balloon effectively to compress the plaque without damaging the artery. Although the technique is no longer considered experimental, the full range of its application is not yet known.

Angioplasty seems to work better on patients in the early stages of atherosclerosis, when the obstructing plaque is still soft enough to be compressed against the

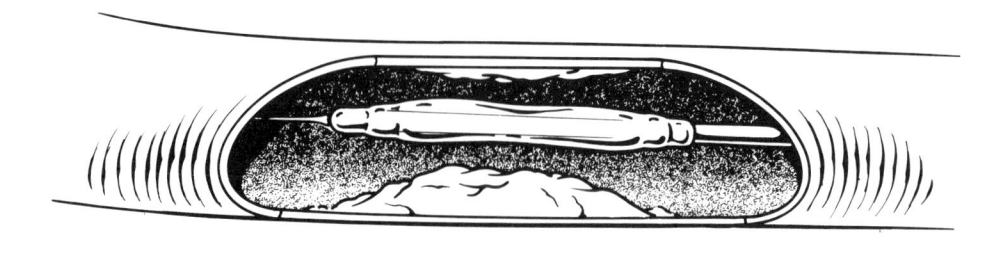

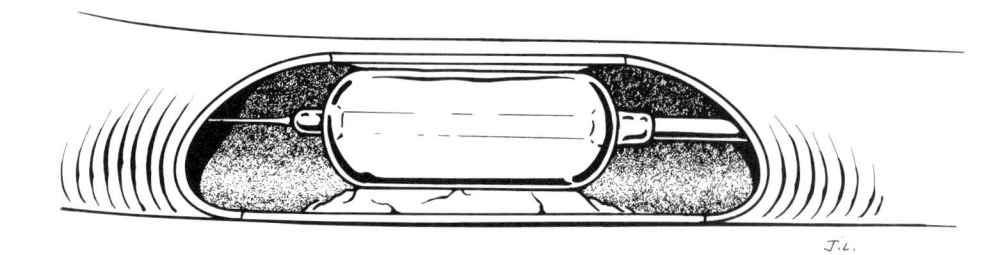

In the procedure called angioplasty, a balloon catheter is threaded into a partially blocked coronary artery (*top*). When the balloon is inflated (*bottom*), it reduces the blockage by compressing the obstructing plaque into the artery wall, opening a larger path for blood flow. As in cardiac catheterization, only a local anesthetic is needed for angioplasty. The patient remains awake and can watch some of the procedure on a screen while it is taking place.

12. What's Ahead in Treating Heart Disease

artery wall. Patients with more advanced cases of coronary artery disease usually have hardened plaque in their arteries, which may crack rather than flatten against the wall. The success rate of angioplasty increases when the physicians at medical centers do a greater number of these procedures. Centers doing fewer than thirty cases a year generally have a success rate of about 65 to 70 percent; busier centers, such as Cleveland Clinic, have a success rate of about 90 percent. Successful angioplasty enlarges the opening in the artery by at least 20 percent, to restore an adequate blood flow to the heart muscle and to eliminate angina pain.

But for many patients, angioplasty does not produce a long-term improvement in their coronary circulation. In many cases, the arteries become obstructed again within six months. Jay Hollman, M.D., a Cleveland Clinic cardiologist who has participated in several thousand angioplasty procedures, says, "Although we are able to fix 90 percent of the patients with angioplasty, we still have a recurrence rate of about 25 percent, which seems to be a standard rate around the country. Most of these recurrences happen within the first six months. And most of the patients who have a recurrence undergo a successful second angioplasty. Of these, only 25 percent will come back with a second recurrence."

Angioplasty is, however, a tempting alternative to coronary bypass surgery for those patients whose condition allows it. Instead of the minimum seven-day hospital stay and six-week recovery period for bypass surgery, angioplasty patients are only in the hospital three days. There is no recuperation from surgery and they can resume a normal, active life immediately. The costs are far less than bypass surgery, as is the time away from work.

However convenient and painless angioplasty is, the procedure is not without risk, since complications can arise during the procedure. Older, calcified plaque may crack and split the artery, slowing blood flow. The artery may go into spasm after the balloon inflates. Occasionally the patient's heart may signal its objection to the intruding catheter by beating erratically.

In cases of cracked arteries with slowed blood flow or arterial spasm, emergency bypass surgery is performed. Whenever a patient is scheduled for angioplasty at the Cleveland Clinic, the cardiac surgeons are alerted and a bed in the cardiac intensive care unit is reserved. Should the patient need immediate bypass surgery, he or she is wheeled from the cardiac catheterization laboratory down the hall into the operating room. Currently, about 5 percent of the angioplasties begun at the Cleveland Clinic culminate in bypass surgery, but this number is expected to drop as continuing research leads to procedures for better identifying the most suitable candidates for angioplasty and the technical problems are solved.

Another exciting possibility for the future is a technique of using laser beams to destroy plaque that blocks arteries. The technique is under intensive developmental

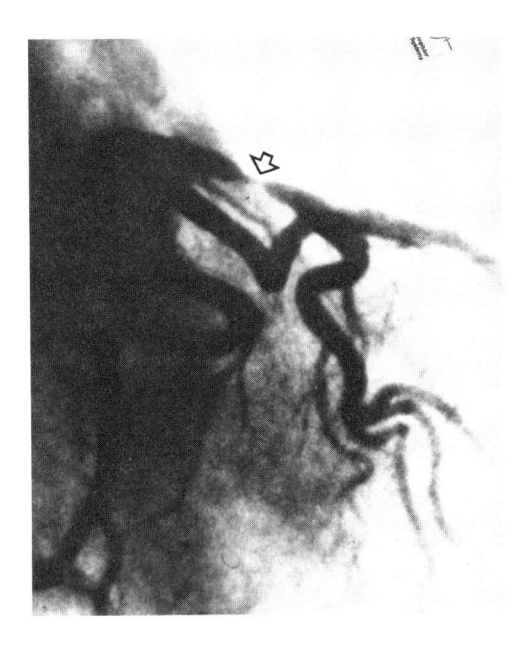

These X-ray pictures of a patient's coronary arteries show a severe obstruction of blood flow in one vessel before angioplasty was performed (*top picture*). After the procedure, blood flow through the same artery is greatly improved (*bottom picture*).

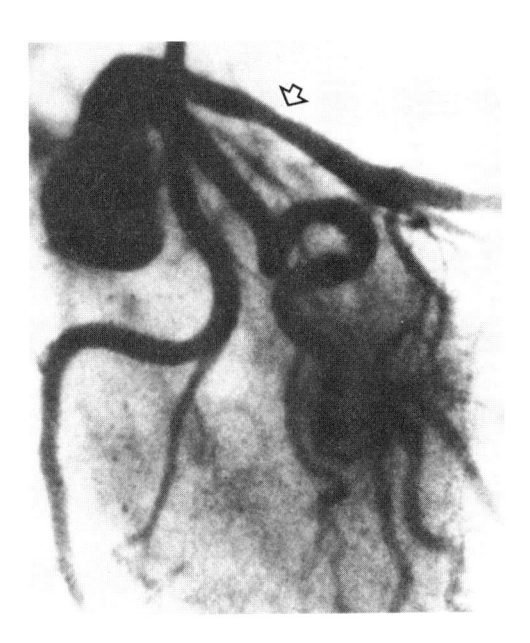

research and testing now, but it may be several years before it is perfected for use. Laser removal of plaque would involve threading a catheter into the coronary artery, just as in cardiac catheterization. Laser light would be beamed through an optical fiber in the catheter to vaporize the blockage in billionth-of-a-second bursts.

To date, the major stumbling block in the development of the technique has been finding a way to destroy the plaque without burning holes in the walls of arteries. Great precision will be needed, and this is where a great deal of emphasis is being placed in research and development. The laser technique has been tested on the arteries of animals and human cadavers. As it is developed further, it will be tested on obstructions of leg vessels in patients.

The era of human heart transplants is now nearly two decades old. These transplants continue to offer hope to desperately ill patients, and probably will until an artificial heart system is perfected. Statistics compiled by the American Heart Association in 1984 showed that eleven medical centers in the United States had at that time performed a total of 635 heart transplants since the first American transplant by Dr. Norman Shumway of Stanford University in 1968. Of that total, 295 patients were still living in 1984 and the one-year survival rate was reported at 80 percent, with estimates for two-year survival projected at about 75 percent.

In the early years of heart transplant operations, the survival rates of heart recipients were disappointingly

12. What's Ahead in Treating Heart Disease

low. They were so disappointing, in fact, that many medical centers stopped doing transplants. To prevent the recipients' bodies from rejecting the foreign tissue of their new hearts, massive doses of immunosuppressant drugs were administered. The drugs left patients with little resistance to infection, and many of them died.

But a new drug, Cyclosporin A, has reduced the frequency of rejection and infection. The number of heart transplants has risen again in recent years and survival rates appear to be improving.

At the same time, the quest for an effective artificial heart has been the focus of dedicated professionals in medical research. The implantation of the Jarvik-7 artificial heart in several patients received national media attention as the doctors performing the operations attempted to learn more about its effects on the human body. To date a major drawback to use of this artificial heart has been the occurrence of strokes in the recipients. The pioneering work will undoubtedly continue in the future.

Other research is being conducted on artificial hearts at different medical centers. The Cleveland Clinic Foundation, for example, has been in the forefront of such research for years through its Department of Artificial Organs, which has been responsible for achievements with artificial hearts, artificial kidneys, artificial lungs, and more recently, artificial livers. The research in this department has been tied to practical benefits for Cleveland Clinic patients, which requires a careful, step-

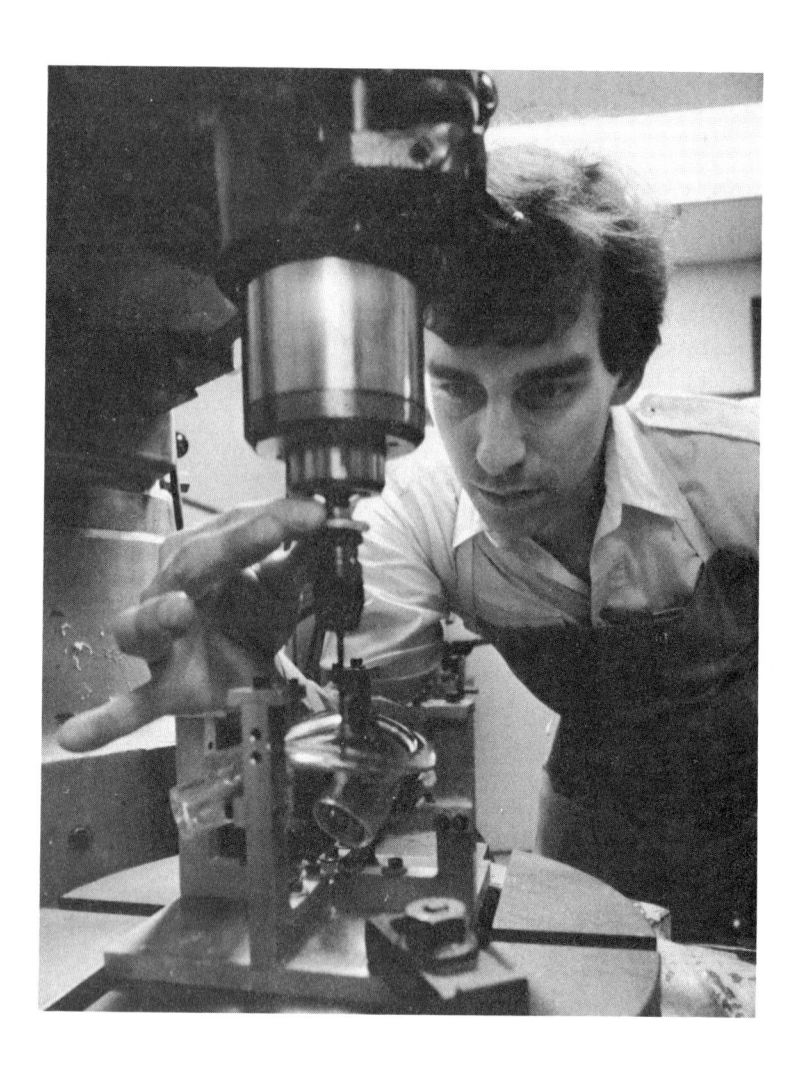

A fabrication technologist at the Cleveland Clinic machines a plastic blood-pump housing for a temporary-assist device that will eventually be used to help heart patients. The Clinic's Department of Artificial Organs has been working for more than a decade to develop heart-assist pumps.

12. What's Ahead in Treating Heart Disease

by-step approach. Clinic researchers have been working on blood pumps to assist the chambers of the heart, as well as entire artificial hearts.

For each patient, they believe the best option should be made available—whether it be temporary pumping while the heart recovers, temporary pumping while waiting for a heart transplant, permanent pumping for one of the heart's pumping chambers (ventricles), or permanent pumping for both ventricles.

"Most people could live very well with one pump to take over the function of the left pumping chamber," explains Leonard A. Golding, M.D., of the Clinic's Department of Thoracic and Cardiovascular Surgery and the Department of Artificial Organs. "But there are some people who would need both sides replaced. Ultimately, once we solve the problems for a single pump, putting in two pumps would be easy.

"That is why to progress sensibly, an artificial heart program must pass through certain phases like testing different advances in animals, changing things when problems arise and finally arriving at what you believe to be a usable device. The best way, then, to introduce the artificial heart in humans is to use it on a temporary basis in carefully selected patients. Meanwhile, experiments in animals continue for longer periods of time, and the technique gradually improves. You put all this experience together, and if you've got a package that fits, you consider permanent implantation."

The Cleveland Clinic Foundation has been following

this format for the past decade or more, during which time its researchers have designed and tested various pumps. Today, several kinds of artificial hearts designed here work efficiently in animals for long periods of time. The U.S. Food and Drug Administration approved the use of the Cleveland Clinic's temporary artificial heart device, which has been used in patients having unusual difficulty recovering from open heart surgery or massive heart attacks.

Researchers here are also working on a permanent artificial heart made of titanium, a lightweight, extremely durable metal used in aircraft, which has been found to be nonreactive in the human body. But concern about the quality of the patient's life after implantation has kept them from implanting it in a human being. They would like to move beyond the present state of artificial heart systems, which require the patient to have chest tubes connected to a cumbersome external power source. The danger of infection here is considerable, so the goal is the implantation of a small, internal power source that would eliminate the tubes and allow the patient to be normally active.

Finding an energy delivery system small enough to fit inside a human chest is an obstacle to overcome. To search for a solution, the Cleveland Clinic has been working under a federal grant to combine its artificial heart pump with internal energy systems being designed at two other centers.

With all these research advances, plus the development

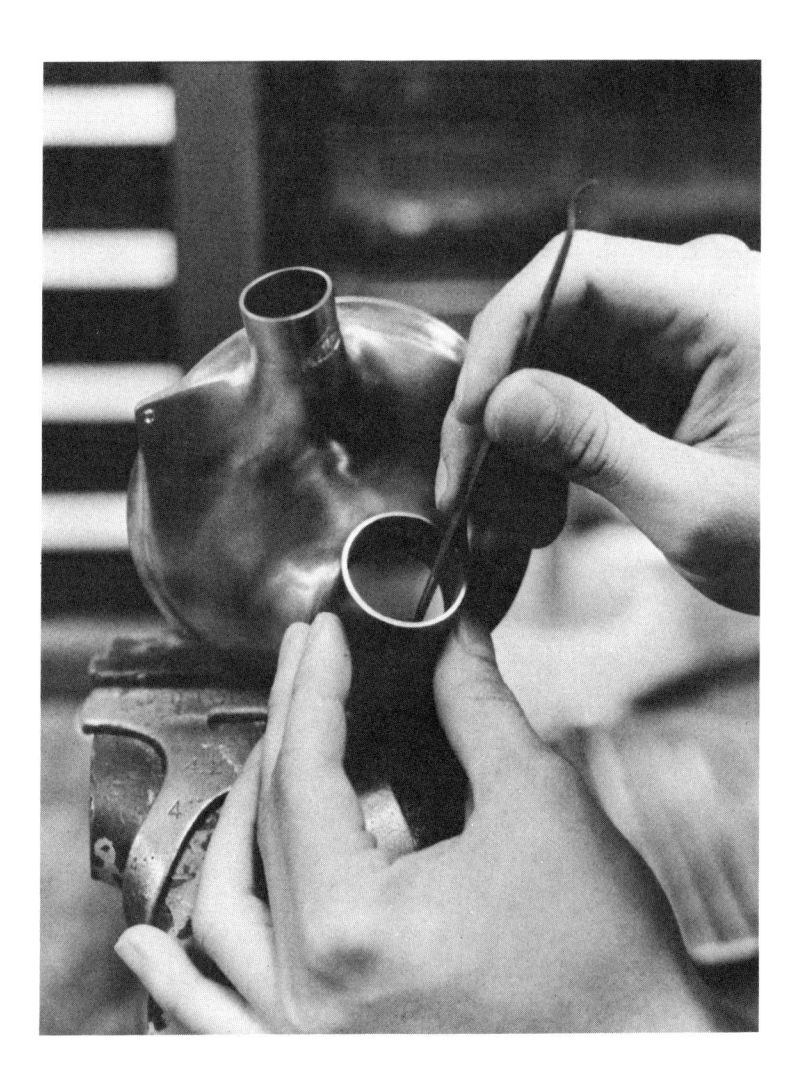

This titanium housing of a left-ventricular-assist blood pump was developed at the Cleveland Clinic. Artificial heart research here is proceeding in several areas, including temporary pumping aid for hearts that are recovering and permanent implantation for patients who need it. The deliberate, step-by-step approach being taken in this research includes experimental implantation in animals.

of new drugs for treating heart disease, heart patients can look forward with hope to the future. And some day, if a way can be found to prevent or reverse heart disease, mankind will be spared the cruelty of one of its most terrible afflictions.

Glossary

angina pectoris, chest pain as the result of inadequate oxygenation of the heart muscle

aorta, the main artery arising from the heart

arrhythmia, a general term for an irregular heartbeat

arteriosclerosis, a disease of arteries in which deposits of cholesterol and other substances in the artery wall can impede the flow of blood

artery, any of a number of blood vessels that carry blood away from the heart to tissues throughout the body

artificial pacemaker, an electrical device that initiates the heartbeat

atherosclerosis, a type of arteriosclerosis that first develops beneath the inner wall of an artery

atrioventricular node, the specialized muscle fibers at the base of the wall between the heart's two upper chambers that act as a relay to conduct the impulse that generates the heartbeat from the atria to the ventricles

atrium, one of the two upper chambers of the heart

autonomic nervous system, the nerves that control such functions as the regulation of heartbeat and the blood pressure, as well as myriad other activities in the body that are not under conscious control blood pressure, the force exerted by the blood against the arteries. See also *hypertension*

bradycardia, an abnormally slow heartbeat

capillary, the smallest blood vessel in which the transfer of oxygen and nutrients to cells takes place

cardiac arrest, cessation of the heartbeat

cardiopulmonary resuscitation, a combination of mouth-to-mouth breathing and heart massage, performed to sustain the circulation of the blood in a person whose heart is beating ineffectively or who is in cardiac arrest

carotid sinus, a small cluster of specialized cells in the carotid arteries that monitors the oxygen and carbon-dioxide content of the blood

cholesterol, a fatlike substance manufactured by cells

coronary arteries, the blood vessels that supply the heart muscle with oxygen and nutrients

coronary bypass, a surgical procedure in which one or more nondiseased vessels, taken from the chest or legs or both, are grafted below the blockage in coronary arteries to keep the heart muscle supplied with blood

coronary occlusion, an obstruction in a coronary artery that shuts off the flow of blood to a portion of the heart muscle. Also called heart attack or myocardial infarction

defibrillator, an electrical device that delivers a shock to the heart

diastole, the phase of the heart's cycle in which the ventricles fill and during which the heart rests for a split second (the "bottom" number in a blood-pressure reading)

Glossary

digitalis, a drug, derived from the foxglove plant, used to stimulate the heart

diuretic, a type of medication used to promote the excretion of urine; often given to treat heart failure or high blood pressure

electrocardiogram (EKG or ECG), the graph of sharp peaks and valleys, usually recorded on a strip of paper, of the heart's electrical impulses; used to help diagnose heart disease.

endocardium, the thin layer of tissue of the inner lining of the heart, in contact with the blood

epicardium, the layer of tissue on the outside of the heart but just inside the pericardium

heart attack, the death of a portion of the heart muscle. See also *myocardial infarction*

heart block, a condition in which the electrical impulse that coordinates the heartbeat is slowed or blocked along its pathway

heart failure, a condition in which the heart is unable to pump enough blood, congestive heart failure

heart-lung machine, a device that diverts the circulation from the heart during surgery. It adds oxygen to the blood, extracts waste gases, and pumps the blood back into the body to support basic life functions while the heart is stilled

heart murmur, an abnormal sound emanating from the heart

hemoglobin, an iron-and-protein complex within red blood cells. It binds oxygen to transport it throughout the body; it binds carbon monoxide even more strongly than oxygen high density lipoprotein (HDL), a normal component of the blood that transports cholesterol

hormone, any of a number of substances that are normally secreted into the circulation by glands

hypertension, high blood pressure

insufficiency, used in conjunction with a specific valve; the incomplete closing of a valve, permitting backflow of blood—as in "mitral insufficiency"

low density lipoprotein (LDL), a normal component of blood that transports cholesterol

mitral valve, two specialized leaflets or cusps of tissue between the left atrium and the left ventricle that permit a one-way flow of blood between those chambers

myocardial infarction (MI), the death of heart muscle by interruption of the blood supply. Sometimes used as a synonym for "heart attack"

nitroglycerin, a drug used to relieve the pain of angina pectoris

pacemaker, a natural or artificial timekeeper for the heartbeat. The body's natural pacemaker is known as the sinoatrial node, a group of cells in the heart that produces the electrical impulses that initiate heart contractions. An electrical pacemaker is a device that substitutes for a defective natural pacemaker by delivering a series of rhythmic electrical discharges to the heart through electrodes. *See also sinoatrial node*

NORMAN V. RICHARDS lives and works in Findlay, Ohio, where he manages the Publications Department for Marathon Oil Company. A former managing editor of *Patient Care*, a national medical journal for family practitioners, he has written twenty-two books and also contributes to magazines on a variety of subjects. In 1982, he underwent open heart surgery at the Cleveland Clinic, an experience which prompted him to write *Heart to Heart*.